The Forgotten Future

The Forgotten Future

Adolescents in Crisis

Deborah Clark Ebel, R.N.

Outskirts Press, Inc.
Denver, Colorado

Outskirts Press, Inc.
http://www.outskirtspress.com

ISBN: 978-1-4327-1935-7

Library of Congress Control Number: 2008921500

Outskirts Press and the "OP" logo are trademarks belonging to Outskirts Press, Inc.

PRINTED IN THE UNITED STATES OF AMERICA

To my parents,

Mildred Luffman French and Roy Howard French,

with love and gratitude

Table of Contents

Author's Note

I came to the field of psychiatric nursing later than many. By the time I graduated from nursing school, I had already born three children, two of whom were still toddlers. Following several years working on a pediatric medical-surgical unit, I joined the staff of a new inpatient adolescent psychiatric unit at the same general hospital. Most of the nurses on that unit were also new to psychiatric nursing, and we learned alongside each other, growing through academic instruction and practical, real-life experiences. I discovered almost immediately that I enjoyed working with troubled youth, and I sought out every learning opportunity available to me. Since that time, I have been fortunate to have worked with children and adolescents in inpatient psychiatric settings in Connecticut, Alaska, and Virginia.

Because the stories I share are from three geographic areas which are distinct in nature, yet similar in practice, I have combined psychiatric facilities in which I have been employed into one composite hospital which I have called Oak Haven Hospital. Again, due to the similarities of policies and procedures, personnel and situations, I have attributed these to Oak Haven.

The patients depicted herein are actual and individual young people with whom I have worked, and their stories are true. They are not composites. These adolescents are some of the young people whose stories and lives I cherish and who will remain with me forever. Names of patients and staff members have been changed to ensure privacy, and in some instances the sequence of events has been changed, solely for purposes of clarity and continuity. I have no idea how many children or teens that I have worked with over the years, and I do not know the outcomes of most of their stories. Many of their names have long since been forgotten to me, but I can still hear their voices … their laughter … their crying.

Because the tragic story of Andrew McClain's death has been widely reported in the news media, I have used the actual names of those involved. Andrew's death played a large part of who I am today and what I think and believe about mental health care for our children.

It has been a privilege to have worked with these young people and an honor to have worked with many of the nurses, doctors, mental health techs, and other mental health workers whose paths have crossed mine. I have been blessed.

Deborah Clark Ebel
Norfolk, Virginia
February, 2008

Introduction

Nightmares have long plagued me. At first they were infrequent, but then they started coming two, sometimes three times a night. Some are terrifyingly real, and I find myself lost, wandering through a surreal Kafkaesque landscape. I recognize others as dreams and awaken disoriented, struggling to free myself from labyrinthine shadows between this world and the other.

Most of the dreams are about kids: kids who have been mistreated, abused, debased, or abandoned. It's never the same dream, except for the kids' pain. In the nightmares, I stand alone, unable to move, riveted in place. Forced to watch as adults destroy kids, as kids destroy kids, as kids destroy themselves. I am helpless to do anything, unable to save anyone.

Some of the kids are runaways; some are throwaways. There are those who have been horribly abused, and many who use drugs or alcohol or sex to avoid confronting the reality of their lives. Others are members or hangers-on of gangs whose perception of normal life includes guns and knives, violence and mayhem. These are the kids I chose to work with, kids who, in many cases, have never before had an adult look them straight in the eye and talk to them about the truths of their lives.

As a registered nurse, I chose to work with teens within a psychiatric setting. I made that decision because our children are the future of our country and because I was, and still am, concerned for all of their tomorrows.

No one ever said working with troubled teens would be easy. I began working with adolescents because I like them. I enjoy being around them. They are enthusiastic and challenging, inquisitive and energetic. They view life with a fresh and idealistic eye. Or at least they used to.

Due to their individual backgrounds and life experiences, an unfortunate number of young people today view life in a jaundiced, hopeless, angry way that in many cases includes violence, substance abuse, self-mutilation, and sexual acting-out. Society's changing values regarding drug use, sexuality, violence in the media, and social structure are adopted, reflected, and then exaggerated by our most vulnerable population: young people with little knowledge or understanding of the consequences their choices can bring.

Nothing shocks them, nothing awes or inspires or excites them. Many have little use for heroes or respect or responsibility. They view authority with disdain and reject any notion of rules, limit setting, or self-discipline.

My perspective is obviously somewhat skewed, as my experience has been with kids in a setting distinct from that of much of the rest of society. My observations on adolescence and family life are, in many cases, profoundly different from what is encountered by most Americans.

I do not mean to imply that these troubled youngsters are typical of our youth. There are millions of children who are able to achieve, despite whatever challenges or obstacles are set before them. These young people approach adulthood with goals and ideals, respect and responsibility.

The young people about whom I am most concerned are those who have become so haunted by what has come before that they have developed into distressed caricatures of their former selves. Many seem to have no sense of what's right or what's wrong, what's good or what's evil, what's honorable and what's without integrity; young people who refuse to accept responsibility for their actions and behavior, who blame others for everything wrong with their lives and value nothing. My concern is for those who, in many cases encouraged by the media, push propriety and good taste to the edge and beyond. I fear for those teens who play a form of Russian roulette with sex, drugs, guns, and lifestyle … and in many cases, lose. If allowed to continue, this downward spiral will take a huge toll on society: financially, socially, medically and morally.

Negative media reports involving children and teenagers are always attention-grabbers, whether the child/teen is portrayed as victim or as perpetrator, and a disturbing picture emerges. The attention is usually temporary, however, as stories are told, studies are done, and fingers are pointed.

While stories and statistics fill volumes, they do not tell all. Numbers do not tell the anguish and devastation in the eyes of a teenager who has been brutally raped by her father and brothers. Numbers do not explain the despair of a gifted teenager so distraught over the hostility and violence in his family that he turns a gun on himself and is left forever functioning at preschool level. Numbers do not explain the lack of remorse in the heart of a young man who callously risks the lives of all around him, solely to meet his own desires.

I have worked with these young people and others—the teenage prostitutes, drug addicts, the despondent, the abandoned—and as I have been touched by each and every one of them, I have come to question our country's priorities. We like to speak of being a child and family-oriented nation, but we're not. No society which allows such atrocities, which tolerates the destruction of childhood, which forgets that *all* children deserve a future, is child-oriented.

While I initially began writing these pages as a sort of catharsis, a way to "vent" and sort out so many emotions after years of working with children and adolescents within the mental health care system, I found the experience to be more difficult than I could ever have imagined. I found myself mentally reliving many of the events and frequently and repeatedly dissolving into tears. There had been so many times on the job that I was unable to permit myself to feel and had to work within the boundaries of my professional role that when I finally allowed myself to take a second look at the situation, it hurt to my very soul.

I found I was able to write for only very short periods. Situations were often too intensely painful for me to think about and put into words beyond considering them for a few minutes at a time. As difficult as it was for me to remember, though, it was even harder for the kids to live. What I most hope to impress upon the reader is that the lives of these young people and the attitudes and behaviors which spring from their experiences are far more commonplace than most have acknowledged or would like to believe. These are not "bad" kids. They are troubled kids. They are our children, every single one of them.

Like much of America, I used to live in a world of smiling, happy, children participating in school field trips, Boy and Girl Scouts, PTA meetings, and birthday parties. A world of kids who went to piano lessons and Saturday afternoon matinees, who had pajama parties and filled out college applications and attended school proms. The world we would all like to imagine for children. The reality, for many, is far from this. We close our eyes to avoid seeing the truth.

My nightmares continue. Perhaps I have allowed too much pain to touch me for too long. Ideally, I should be objective and distance myself from the situations I encounter without losing my concern for the kids. I suppose I could intellectualize or give less of myself, but would that help? I don't think so. I have looked into their souls and seen their pain. I know we have let so many of them down. We gave them life, yet by not meeting the needs of our young, we are sacrificing their future.

It's time that we reestablish our roles as mentors, teachers, nurturers, healers; time to reach out and join hands and do our jobs as real adults and as children have a right to expect.

Our children's future must not be forgotten.

Chapter 1
The Fourth Floor

The imposing fieldstone building might easily be mistaken for an Old Guard estate, were it not for the small, discretely-placed sign declaring one's arrival at Oak Haven Hospital. Nestled among centuries-old oaks, the hospital has co-existed amicably, albeit at arm's length, with its residential neighbors for some twenty-five years.

During the summer, the grounds are ablaze with flowering plants and shrubs of every imaginable size and description. In winter, the snow-covered hills recall gentler times when woolen-clad boys and girls skimmed toboggans over adjacent hills. It's a peaceful image, a place where many seek safety and refuge and healing. Where some recover their lost selves. Where still others wreak havoc with the system and with themselves.

A place where reality is not always as it appears to the outsider.

Once inside the main building, staff and visitors looking westward from the uppermost floor have an expansive view of the river with its vintage suspension bridge. The bridge itself is the subject of countless local rumors concerning former Oak Haven patients who have taken their lives by plunging from one of its towers. In fact, in the seventy-plus years since the bridge was constructed, only one suicide has been completed from the bridge, and that was in 1956, long before the existence of Oak Haven.

The facts notwithstanding, locals freely engage in the telling and retelling of their ignoble tales without much concern for the truth. In the world of Oak Haven, however, reality is often stranger than the stuff of imagination.

Oak Haven is one of the hundreds of state and private psychiatric hospitals and community hospital psychiatric units in the United States. Although the hospital is small by some measures, Oak Haven's services are comparable to those of larger facilities in the range of services offered. Inpatient hospitalization is available for children, pre-teens, adolescents, and adults, as is more specific inpatient treatment for those adolescent and adult patients with substance abuse issues. Outpatient counseling is available for all of the above, and community service programming is provided, although with only limited success.

Treatment at Oak Haven is expensive. Figures are not quoted directly, but charges in excess of $1,000 per patient per day are typical. Commercial insurance is eagerly accepted, as are self-pay, Medicaid, and Tricare payments. Unfortunately, if the prospective patient is not covered by one of these payment options, he or she must obtain treatment elsewhere.

Over and above the basic rate, patients are charged for each item provided, from a bulk-purchase, hard-bristle toothbrush, to a small box of tissues, to a package of sanitary pads, to the composition books in which patients complete their journal assignments. There are no freebies at Oak Haven.

Inpatient treatment in America's psychiatric hospitals is designated as either *voluntary* or *involuntary*. More than a patient's or family's preference, these are legal status distinctions determined by a licensed physician or judicial official.

A designation of *voluntary* indicates the patient acknowledges the need for immediate placement within a hospital setting and agrees to participate in the services provided by the hospital. Services offered usually include group and individual therapy, occupational therapy, recreation therapy, and specialty groups such as those for post traumatic stress disorder (PTSD), substance abuse treatment, detox, or other. No legal entity has ordered or required the hospitalization, and these patients are permitted to leave when they choose with proper notice to the hospital.

An *involuntary* patient is one who has been remanded to the custody of the psychiatric hospital for a specified period of time because he or she has been determined to pose an immediate danger to himself or herself or others, is unable to care for himself or herself, or is deemed to be "gravely disabled". These patients must remain in the hospital until a doctor determines that the patient is safe to leave or until further judicial determination is made. This is what is commonly referred to as being *committed*. Each state has its own criteria regarding commitment.

Oak Haven's primary orientation is toward the voluntary population, although there is a ten-bed close observation unit (COU) for acutely suicidal or homicidal patients who are usually involuntarily-committed. While there exist psychiatric facilities where patients are held for an indefinite period of time, all of Oak Haven's units are considered short term; that is, hospitalization generally lasts from two to six weeks. There are, however, situations in which patients leave after 24 hours or remain for several months.

Being a voluntary patient, however, doesn't always mean *voluntary*, especially in the case of adolescents. That's where things can really get confusing. For the most part, the kids don't want any part of being in the hospital and are there only because their parents and doctors have compelled them. Despite widespread belief (on the part of the young patients) to the contrary, there is no commitment on them and no official hold. If the parents and the child's psychiatrist agree that the child is safe for discharge, this can usually be done without any formality beyond that involved in a regular discharge from any hospital.

People who work in psychiatric settings deal with situations and behaviors that on the whole make society uncomfortable. Moods encountered among patients during a single shift can vary from frantic euphoria to such abysmal depression that life longs for death. Staff members hear horrific tales of abuse, neglect, and atrocities so evil it shocks to the core and are witness to behaviors so abhorrent that one has to fight the urge to recoil.

Deborah Clark Ebel, R.N.

Working with such a population means being confronted on a daily basis with the pain and turmoil of a dozen or more seriously troubled human beings, and because each of us carries into adulthood our own experiences, fears, triumphs, tragedies, prejudices, and emotional reactions, it can sometimes be difficult for staff members to maintain a balance between therapeutic concern and emotional detachment. Many people begin working in such a setting only to discover after a very short time that the intensely stressful psychiatric environment is more than they bargained for. Working within such an environment requires that one be emotionally healthy and possess the desire to act as support to others, while at the same time be able to avoid being drawn into what are, at times, excruciatingly painful situations.

People who choose to work with adolescents within a psychiatric setting are a special breed. The egocentrism and rebelliousness of normal adolescence compounded by abuse or neglect require that those working with these young people have a special commitment to, and belief in, the future. Facing an out-of-control teenager's anger, hostility, violence, and lack of consideration or regard for the rights or feelings of others can be demoralizing at best and devastating at worst. Listening to, and caring for, an adolescent whose life has been destroyed by the family who should have loved her, or to the young person who believes life's only solution is death, can break even the hardest heart.

Working within such intimacy means laughter, tears, happiness, sorrow, pain, and bearing witness to horrors of the mind so deep that sometimes one wonders if recovery is even possible. It also sometimes means being part of healing a soul and soaring to rapturous heights. We see the worst, and the best, that humanity has to offer.

*   *   *   *

In 1999, the Surgeon General estimated that twenty percent of America's children have mental disorders with at least mild functional impairment. Between six and nine million children under the age of eighteen are said have a *serious* emotional disturbance.

The Forgotten Future

The increasing willingness to acknowledge mental illness as a problem for the young, accompanied by the resulting dramatic increase in the number of diagnoses and psychiatric hospitalizations, has resulted in a change in the types and severity of behaviors for which young people are hospitalized. Even as recently as the 1990s, facilities typically dealt more with runaways, depression, adolescent behavior problems, and moderate levels of drug and alcohol use. The long-term care mentally ill patients, the hard-core or violent patients, and those with legal involvement were usually sent to public or state-run institutions for longer periods of care. Today, however, a significant number of young people in private facilities have been engaged in illegal and/or violent activities and are in some way involved with the juvenile justice system.

There are systemic problems with psychiatric hospitalization as it exists today, and those problems interfere with our children receiving the treatment they need and deserve. Patients suffering from what are termed "mood disorders" (i.e., major depression, dysthymia, bipolar disorder, etc.,) and "anxiety disorders" (such as panic disorders, phobias, agoraphobia, post-traumatic stress disorder, etc.), as well as patients exhibiting more overt and negative behaviors (diagnoses such as impulse-control disorders, including conduct disorder, oppositional defiant disorder, substance abuse, antisocial behavior, and others), are routinely housed and treated together. This frequently results in situations wherein the needs of neither group are adequately met. Many of those who have engaged in the more severe negative behaviors have not only consciously chosen to participate in their activities, but desire to continue doing so.

Not infrequently, young people in hospitals who could benefit from intensive mental health services do not receive optimal care simply because many of their peers demand more aggressive care and intervention. The old adage "the squeaky wheel gets the grease" is certainly true here. Acting-out and behaviorally-disordered youth require an inordinate amount of staff time and attention, time and attention that could, and should, be spent working with those who truly desire help with their problems.

While confronting that reality, it's important to understand that there are usually underlying reasons why some young people exhibit such negative behavior and attitudes—in most cases they have not chosen such devastating master plans for their lives. We cannot presume to accurately gauge the extent of harm done to a child or adolescent by physical, sexual, emotional or verbal abuse or neglect, or any other situation a child might have experienced, and because we cannot fully understand how an individual child might respond following difficult life circumstances, we are often unable to recognize the extreme hurt behind their negative behavior or accept that their "bad" behavior is rooted in harm done to the child.

Therein lies the dichotomy, the confusion, the frustration inherent in working with troubled adolescents. As human beings, we have an immediate desire to recoil, to pull away, to protect ourselves from those whose behavior is so out-of-control that their actions cause enormous turmoil and pain to others. We want to shield ourselves and, by extension, our loved ones from the disruption and destruction caused by these youth.

At the same time, despite any negative feelings we may experience toward those in our care, mental health professionals have a need to *understand,* and we desperately want to show compassion, no matter the presenting behavior or problem. We want to teach and encourage positive values and provide comfort and facilitate healing,

Healing. It's always about the healing.

With that in mind, a look at the presenting problems of teenagers hospitalized in a particular private institution on a typical and random day showed the following:

Jason is fourteen and has been diagnosed with major depression and attention deficit hyperactivity disorder (ADHD). He has had numerous previous psychiatric admissions, and his history includes having been violently raped at the age of eleven by members of a street gang. He admits to sexually molesting younger children of both sexes as well as the regular use of marijuana and alcohol. He has assaulted school staff, lies regularly, and has been known to steal frequently. On our inpatient unit, he was placed on sexual acting out precautions.

The Forgotten Future

Zeke is thirteen and has been diagnosed with adjustment disorder and ADHD. Four days prior to admission, he choked a friend at school after the friend "looked at (him) the wrong way". He has a long history of physical and verbal assault on peers and staff at school and was suspended twice in the first four months of the school year. He has been barred from neighborhood youth clubs due to his behavior. He admits to using alcohol and marijuana regularly, and LSD and cocaine occasionally. He has had numerous previous psychiatric admissions.

Phil is fourteen and has been diagnosed with conduct disorder and polysubstance abuse. He is heavily involved with street gangs and has a history of assaulting school staff and peers. He began smoking cigarettes at age ten and now admits to using marijuana and alcohol on a regular basis.

James is fourteen and has been diagnosed with adjustment disorder, dysthymia, and polysubstance abuse. On the day of admission, he assaulted both a female teacher and another student at school. The police report states he threw the teacher to the ground and began to strangle her. She was rescued by the school's custodian who reportedly "beat" the patient off. He has had numerous previous psychiatric admissions.

Jared is fourteen and has been diagnosed with conduct disorder. Several weeks prior to admission he threatened to kill an acquaintance at school. The other male learned of his plan and attacked the patient first, beating him in the head with a hammer. When authorities arrived, the patient was found to have in his possession an eleven-inch lug wrench with which he apparently planned to kill the other male. He is now fixated on obtaining a sawed-off twelve-gauge shotgun to "shoot the bastard in the face". He had previously been expelled from school for carrying a concealed weapon and is known to participate in the manufacture and sale of methamphetamine. There is heavy gang involvement. The patient is from an intact family and has no history of emotional, physical, or sexual abuse.

Kendra is fourteen and has been diagnosed with depression and bulimia. Prior to admission, she attempted suicide for the second time by swallowing 100 antibiotic pills. The patient is from an intact family in which her father is a policeman and her mother is a homemaker. She has no history of emotional, physical, or sexual abuse.

Zoe is a sixteen-year-old female, diagnosed with oppositional defiant disorder. She has run away from home numerous times and was most recently stopped as she attempted to board a plane to another state. After being returned home by the police, she trashed her house, breaking furniture and spray-painting the living room. She was suspended from school twice in the first four months of the school year. She was adopted at the age of three days by a family that remains intact. There is no history of emotional, physical, or sexual abuse.

Travis is fourteen and has been diagnosed with major depression, ADHD, and oppositional defiant disorder. He admits to being suspended from school five times, running away twice, skipping school countless times, vandalizing property twice, drinking alcohol numerous times, shoplifting once, and fighting six times. He is known to lie frequently, and the numbers given for his infractions are believed to be gross under-exaggerations. He is reported to be hanging out with "peers of negative influence".

Sixteen-year-old Alicea has been diagnosed with depression and polysubstance abuse. Prior to admission, she took an overdose of 175 aspirin in her second suicide attempt; two weeks prior to this, she threatened to shoot herself, but a friend took the gun away and threw it into a dumpster. She admits to the use of alcohol and marijuana since the age of twelve.

Bonnie, thirteen, has been diagnosed with polysubstance abuse, major depression, and oppositional defiant disorder. She admits to frequent thoughts of suicide and has numerous scars all over her body from self-inflicted cuts and lighter burns.

Heather, fourteen, has been diagnosed with major depression. Her history includes her arrest following the theft of a friend's mother's ATM card and its use to obtain several thousand dollars from the victim's savings account. She has also reportedly stolen an expensive digital camera, a 22-caliber gun, and jewelry. She regularly hangs out with an eighteen-year-old known drug dealer and admits to the frequent use of marijuana and alcohol. She also admits to selling drugs. She feels no remorse for her actions and believes she has done nothing wrong; indeed, she states the victims were so careless with their possessions that they themselves were responsible for the thefts. Her mother is currently in prison for selling drugs.

Janida is sixteen and has been diagnosed with major depression. She reports having felt suicidal for the past two years. She refuses to speak to, or about, her family. She states she is a "black witch" who sees and speaks to demons and monsters. She studies witchcraft and reportedly casts evil spells on her enemies and enjoys frightening peers with tales of her "powers".

*   *   *   *

When considering mental health care and psychiatric hospitalization, the public tends to think of and credit the medical staff and, in particular, the psychiatrists, for the changes effected in patients with successful outcomes. The reality is that hospitalized patients who have actual contact with a physician every day of their stay are the exception, as are those who have daily contact with a psychiatric social worker or psychologist. Occupational therapists, recreation therapists, and substance abuse educators may also see patients one or more times a week.

The nursing staff, however, is responsible for and monitors patients twenty-four hours a day, seven days a week. Working eight- or twelve-hour shifts, frequently without the benefit of even a meal or bathroom break, is, in many ways, analogous to living with the patients. We see their ups and downs, their mood changes, their reactions to significant as well as insignificant events. We see their responses to medication, stressful events, and challenges to their behaviors. We monitor their use of effective and ineffective coping skills and their manner and style of communicating. We receive their affection and their hostility, their indifference and their anger.

In many ways, we do the same with doctors. We see their ups and downs, their mood changes, their reactions to significant as well as insignificant events, their responses to stressful events, and challenges to their directives. We monitor their use of effective and ineffective coping skills and their manner and style of communicating. We receive their praise and their hostility, their indifference and their anger. We deal with their personalities and idiosyncrasies and respond in whatever way will most help our patients.

*   *   *   *

Meghan stomped off the elevator and glared at me with a look that begged the opportunity to verbally destroy me. At fifteen, she already wore the look of an angry and embittered young woman who has seen life from its underbelly. We hadn't even met yet, and she had already decided I was the enemy

"Hi! My name is Debbi." I smiled and extended my hand. "I'm one of the nurses here on the adolescent unit."

Meghan gave me a weak I-couldn't-care-less handshake and continued to glare. "I'm Meghan," she replied after a long pause. "That's M-E-G-H-A-N. Meghan with an 'H'."

"Okay, Meghan-with-an-H, welcome!" She wanted to make sure we knew who she was, that she was *someone*. I kept smiling.

When a new patient arrived on the unit, we usually received only very limited information from the admitting crisis worker. Brief details regarding events precipitating the admission and general information on previous therapy were all that could be expected. The patient's history came in bits and pieces over the next several days, gathered from the patient, his or her parents, the psychiatrist, outside sources, and psychological and educational testing. Eventually all this comes together to form a thorough picture of what has happened in the young person's life to bring him or her to this point.

All I knew about Meghan when she arrived on the unit was her name, her age, and that she had been involved in a violent fight with her mother. I also knew she had never been psychiatrically hospitalized before and hadn't even been in therapy.

She didn't speak as we walked down the hall to the conference room. I unlocked the door, and we went in and sat on opposite sides of the long wooden table. We chatted informally—actually, *I* did most of the talking—to give her a few minutes to acclimate herself. Those first minutes gave me a good opportunity to assess her emotional state. I watched her closely—eyes, hand movements, tilt of her head, manner and tone of speech.

"Meghan, you're here on Oak Haven's adolescent mental health unit, and right now there are fourteen kids here, not counting you. It's a mix of boys and girls … the youngest right now is twelve and the oldest is seventeen." I continued with my spiel, a patter that could almost be done by rote.

One of the things I was looking for as I talked was her receptivity or resistance to the situation. Was she amenable to being here? Would she try to run from the unit? Was she at risk for self-mutilation or possibly even suicide? Were the other kids or staff at risk of any harm from Meghan and what did she hope to gain from being here in the hospital? Was she here because she wanted help or because someone made her come?

She didn't ask questions about the unit or even what would happen during her stay, which was not surprising. First-timers are usually scared and, in some cases, expect to see other patients climbing the walls. Literally. Although she fidgeted with the zipper on her coat, she seemed comfortable enough, and we moved ahead with the interview.

"Can you tell me what happened to bring you to the hospital today?" I knew she had been in a fight with her mother, but I wanted to hear her side of things.

"Me and my mom got in a big fight and she brought me here." Meghan wouldn't look at me, but instead looked around the room at everything else: the window, the pictures, the file cabinet, the telephone. Everything except me. She sounded defensive and angry. At her mom, at me, at the world.

I waited for her to continue, but when she didn't, I prompted, "Can you tell me what you were fighting about?"

"Yeah, well, I guess. She was hittin' my little brother, Tyler, you know? Hittin' him in the face like this …" She made several slapping motions with her hand, and her voice rose slightly in pitch and tempo. "She just kept hittin' him, and he was cryin' and stuff. He's just a little baby, he's just one years old, and she wouldn't quit. I told her to stop, and when she didn't, I stepped up and made her. Then her and me started fightin'. That's how I got these bruises. See?" She looked at me briefly and then pulled up her sleeves to show several black and blue marks on her right arm and a couple on her left. She didn't mention the older, resolving bruise on her left cheek.

We spent the next half-hour together, talking and getting to know each other. Meghan visibly relaxed as she realized I wasn't going to challenge or criticize her. She told me that her mom had left their home when Meghan was three years old and that she had been raised primarily by her aging grandmother. Every couple of years her mother would give birth to a new child and drop the baby off to be cared for by the grandmother. Her mother passed into and out of their lives as she pleased, without explanation or excuse.

I learned that her mom worked as a prostitute, making just enough to support herself in a tiny, rundown efficiency apartment. On those rare occasions when she was feeling particularly maternal toward her children and returned to their lives for a brief time, she would take her children to "work" with her. Meghan and her younger brothers and sisters had an early exposure to their mother's service-for-hire business. At this point in time, whether fortunately or unfortunately, her mother had decided she wanted her five children to live with her.

"When I was at my grandma's, y'know, I had to take care of all the little kids. She didn't like to hear 'em be noisy or play too loud, so I had to watch 'em all the time when she was resting. My grandma drinks, so, uh, I had to do the housework, too, and some-times wash her up when she puked. Oh, and I cooked, too."

"Ummm." I nodded my understanding. "Sounds like you pretty much took care of the whole house." I made a couple of notes on the assessment form. I realized that Meghan had become, as do many children in similar households, parentified. "That must've been hard for you ..."

She quickly interjected, "Oh! I didn't mind. It was my job. I like takin' care of little kids."

Like many other youngsters who assume adult responsibilities, she took a certain measure of pride in her abilities and in being "needed". At the same time, I suspected she was keenly aware of having been deprived of any sort of real childhood. I made a mental note of the very worn and ragged purple stuffed Barney sticking out of her backpack.

The interview would have gone further, but Caitlyn opened the door and peeked in. "Sorry to interrupt, but, uh, we have a little problem out here. Could I see you for a minute, Deb?"

"Yep, we were just about through here anyway." I pushed my chair back. "Meghan, come on with me. I'm going to park you down by the nurses' office for a few minutes while I talk to Caitlyn, and then we'll get you settled in your room. We'll finish talking later, okay?"

We both stood, and I let Meghan walk out the door ahead of me. While I truly loved working with the kids, I had long ago learned the hard way never to turn my back on one.

Caitlyn, one of the unit's most conscientious MHTs (mental health tech—an unlicensed aide who is an integral part of any inpatient mental health unit, also sometimes called a mental health counselor or mental health worker) was waiting when I walked into the nurses' office.

"What's up?" I asked as I tapped the loose assessment papers into a neat stack and laid them on the desk.

"Dea says she took some pills yesterday," Caitlyn replied.

"Where in the world did she get pills?" My mind raced with everything that would have to be done if it were true: calls to the doctors, supervisors and parents, laboratory tests, various forms of documentation, and a room search to look for anything else Dea might have.

It seemed as if one or another of the kids was always trying to put something over on the staff, and they frequently came up with imaginative and innovative ideas. For example, one of my former patients, a fifteen-old girl who was into self-mutilation, sneaked in rock-salt from the icy winter sidewalk and used it to burn her arms. The burns were something none of us knew could be done, so we had not anticipated or expected it. But we immediately learned a valuable lesson.

I had known Dea for a long time and I knew she didn't always tell the truth. Sometimes she said things just to manipulate and get attention. I moved toward the nurses' office door. "Did she say what they were?"

"Jackie's in talking to her now. Dea said she brought the pills back with her after pass on Sunday, but she won't say what they were. She told Amber about it this morning, and Amber told Jackie a few minutes ago." Jackie was an excellent MHT who occasionally worked on the adolescent unit.

"Well, I'm gonna go see how Jackie's doing and if she needs anything. Would you do a clothing search and have Meghan change into pajamas and then get a set of vitals on her?" I started down the hall, calling back over my shoulder, "Check through her belongings carefully, okay?"

Dea was sixteen and on her fifth admission to Oak Haven. She had been admitted this time with diagnoses of borderline personality disorder and PTSD after having been gang-raped while attending a college football game. When I walked into her room, she was sitting cross-legged on the bed. Jackie stood by the window, looking more than a little perturbed.

"Thank God you're here," Dea moaned as she rose from the bed with arms outstretched to give me a hug. "She won't listen to me at all." Dea waved her hand dismissively toward Jackie.

"Dea, I'm *listening*. You're just not telling me anything." Jackie sounded exasperated. I knew she was really trying to work with Dea, but things apparently weren't going well.

Adolescents diagnosed with borderline personality disorder see people in their lives as either all good or all bad. They lack the ability to integrate all the aspects of another's personality into a whole and, as a result, see everything as an extreme: good-bad, black-white, love-hate, right-wrong. There is no middle ground, and it's difficult to figure out where they're coming from and what they expect at any given time. They often have difficulty distinguishing between reality (the world as it really is) and their own beliefs (their misperceptions) about the world and their environment.

Early in my nursing career, I had been flattered when a girl who was diagnosed with borderline personality disorder told me I was her "favorite" and that I was the "best" nurse she had ever had. I

The Forgotten Future

was knocked off my pedestal a short while later when she told me she hated me and would never speak to me again because I had placed her on room restriction for shoving another girl.

Dea linked her arm through mine and flashed a smug grin in Jackie's direction. "Why would I tell you anything? You're such a bitch. Debbi is my favorite—I can talk to her 'cause I trust her." She squeezed my arm as she spoke.

She was trying to *split staff,* a favorite pastime of a lot of our kids—especially those with borderline traits—and I had to call her on it. I slipped my arm out of Dea's and motioned her toward her bed. "Dea, I know that sometimes it's easier to talk to one person instead of another, but that's not your choice now. When you brought pills onto this unit, you lost your right to choose who you talk to. What you did was serious, and we need to know all the details." I pulled out the desk chair and sat down, nodding toward Jackie. "And since Jackie was in here talking with you first, she's in charge."

Dea sat in the middle of her bed, carefully arranging the bed pillows before answering. She was obviously considering her options and the repercussions of each before deciding what to say. There was silence for a full thirty seconds or so before she looked up at Jackie and said, "Well all right, I'll tell you. But I'm only talkin' because Debbi is here. I still don't like *you.*" She scrunched up her face at Jackie for emphasis.

I could imagine what kind of response Jackie would have liked to make, but she simply smiled and said, "That's okay, Dea. I'm glad you trust someone enough to tell the truth."

Dea nestled down within her cushioned fortress and smoothed the cover of the pillow on her lap. "I brought in some pills and took 'em, that's all." She shrugged as if to add *no big deal.*

Jackie took the lead and asked, "What kind of pills were they? And how many and when did you take them?"

I remembered from previous admissions that both Dea and her mom had been in the mental health system for a long time, and I could guess she probably had a variety of pills at home, ranging from antidepressants to tranquilizers to who-knows-what. Still, if she took the pills yesterday, she had experienced no overt reaction.

In any case, I'd have to call the medical doctor and, depending on what she took, get some lab tests done. Problems caused by medication—even over-the-counter-medication—are not always immediately apparent.

"Just some aspirins." She stared steadily at Jackie. "I took ten aspirins, that's all."

"Aspirin? Ten aspirin? You didn't take anything else? No Haldol or Ativan or Oxycontin? Nothing besides aspirin?" Jackie wasn't convinced.

"No, I didn't take nothin' else," she answered sarcastically. "Just the aspirins. I'm not stupid, y'know. I didn't really want to hurt myself. I just wanted to see if I could bring pills back with me in case I needed 'em. And I did." She looked away and smiled faintly while continuing to smooth the top of the pillow. "You can run a drug test on me if you want, but the only thing that'll show up is the aspirins."

"So, how did you get the aspirin in? I know we searched your things when you came back from pass, because I was there." The kids often enjoyed bragging after the fact, and maybe this time I could learn a new hiding place for contraband. No matter how carefully we searched, there are always ways to get forbidden items past staff and that could be dangerous for everyone.

"It was easy." Dea got up and sashayed into the bathroom, returning with an open package of sanitary pads. "In here." She thrust the package into my hands and walked back to her bed. "It was easy."

What she was saying didn't register because whenever a patient came back from a pass we always, at the very least, visually inspected the inside of any open package. Maybe we weren't being as thorough as we thought we were. What if she had brought in something more lethal than a few aspirin? I just didn't get it.

"How were they in here?" I asked.

She was already beginning to tire of the game. She jumped up and grabbed the package from my hands, taking out one of the individually wrapped pads. "In here. Inside here," she answered, jabbing her finger into the pad. She was growing impatient and raised her voice ever so slightly. "I unwrapped the pad, ripped a hole in the side, and put the pills in. Then I closed the wrapper back up again. You guys are so stupid, you didn't even look." She tossed the pad onto my lap and sauntered back to her bed. She sat on the bed's edge, looking enormously self-satisfied. "It's easy to bring stuff back in here."

I knew then she had just been testing us to see what she could get away with and we had failed. She had outsmarted us this time, and she was right: anyone with imagination could sneak in just about anything without our knowing, no matter how thorough we tried to be.

* * * *

With a round, cherubic face that would forever belie his age, Dr. Paul Evans looked barely old enough to be out of college, let alone a practicing psychiatrist. His low-keyed rebelliousness expressed itself most openly in his style of dress: his avoidance of the traditional doctor suit and tie for the more casual look of jeans and open-neck cotton shirt. The older docs had at first encouraged him to wear *de rigueur* attire, but they eventually gave up and came to look beyond his appearance and accept him as the skilled practitioner he was.

Dr. Evans avoided the typical psycho-babble when talking with patients and parents, and he patiently listened to their questions and concerns and willingly provided answers in easy-to-understand language. Although unconventional at times, he had a good grasp of the challenges facing many of today's adolescents, and he was respected by just about everyone with whom he came in contact.

Evans had a particularly strong therapeutic relationship with a young man named Daniel. Daniel was fourteen, quickly closing in on thirty, and had recently concluded a successful career as a drug dealer. Following their parents' divorce, Daniel and his sister had been raised by their father, a man with no interest in parenting two children.

Daniel learned early on that he couldn't depend on his father. When Daniel was six years old, he was picked up and sexually assaulted by two adult males and then dumped back out on the street. When he arrived home after dark, scared and crying, and told his dad about the attack, his father's response was to beat him with a belt for being late for supper.

With this as a model for male relationships and behavior, Daniel avoided anything more than minimal interaction with males for the next eight years. He fell into the regular use of alcohol and just about every type of illegal substance available, including the use of heroin a dozen or more times. As a means of supporting his habit, he sold drugs to the eager population of his small college town and was successful enough to enjoy an extensive wardrobe, electronics, and jewelry collection. He looked good, was polished, and could easily have passed for one of his college-age customers.

In reality, he was fourteen, hurt, scared, and very lonely.

One night, during a fight, Daniel threatened to kill his father. Neighbors called the police, and Daniel was promptly arrested and sent to the state juvenile detention facility where he was confined for several months. Upon his release, he and his sister were both shipped off to live with their mother, whom they hadn't seen in years. Suddenly having two teenagers arrive on her doorstep, both of whom were accustomed to leading their own lives, was more than Daniel's mother could handle. Arguments led to threats. Threats led to running away. And running away led Daniel to Oak Haven.

Daniel had been at Oak Haven for about three weeks when he and Evans stopped by the nurses' office one evening. Evans offhandedly announced he was taking Daniel to the main hospital cafeteria.

"We just finished talking, and I thought we'd go grab a bite to eat." Evans picked through the remains of a box of chocolates and passed several through the door to Daniel. "Put these in your pocket for later, and I'll be right out."

Daniel eagerly accepted the candies and then walked over to the hallway bulletin board and stood looking over the notices.

"Are you asking to take him or telling us he's going?" inquired Caitlyn, grabbing the last chocolate from the box.

The Forgotten Future

"I'm telling, but at least I *am* telling. I'm a quick learner." Evans winked at Caitlyn. He had the annoying habit of taking kids off the unit without letting the nursing staff know and leaving us to search the entire unit for a possible runaway only to find Evans had taken the patient to the gift shop, the cafeteria, or for a walk outside. Evans enjoyed spending time with his patients and had been known to order in pizza, have dinner with them in the hospital cafeteria, play games on the unit, even shoot hoops with them at gym time. His style was very different from that of many of the other doctors who often acted as if the kids were an inconvenience.

"Dr. Evans," said Caitlyn, "about that candy you just slipped to Daniel? You know the kids aren't allowed to have it and you do this all the time."

Evans stood and walked toward the door. "Yeah, well, what can I say? I do what I do," He smiled and unlocked the unit door, and he and Daniel walked off toward the cafeteria.

*   *   *   *

Michael was smooth. He said he wanted to be a lawyer when he got older. He was smart and talked a good talk. He also used drugs. *Lots* of drugs.

Michael was admitted to Oak Haven after his third suspension for smoking pot on school grounds. He had been seeing Dr. Evans for several years, but things weren't getting any better for him. Raised by their alcoholic mother, Michael and his twin brother, Matt, had done well in school early on, and both had a desire to someday get out of their not-quite-slum-but-close-to-it neighborhood.

Growing up, Michael and Matt were extremely close to their mother and often assumed a caretaking role, both of their mother and of each other. Inseparable in their early years as twins often are, they remained close until junior high school when each began to develop disparate interests. Michael wanted to study law; Matt wanted to be a teacher. Michael began to drink and party. Matt wasn't interested in the high life, preferring instead to participate on a couple of after-school sports teams.

Their father had abandoned the family when the boys were small, and even though their mother had been involved with several men over the years, there was no consistent authority figure, no male role model, for the boys. Michael began to rebel; Matt began to look at how he could live his life more responsibly than had their father.

I met Michael during his fourth psychiatric admission. He had been admitted twice to other facilities and once previously to Oak Haven before I began working there. During his earlier admission to Oak Haven, he was an angry eleven-year-old who was already beginning to show significant defiance regarding rules.

With a diagnosis of bipolar disorder, sixteen-year-old Michael was supposed to be maintained on lithium. He didn't like the way it made him feel though, so he stopped taking it. When the feelings of depression moved back in, those feelings of loneliness and abandonment, those feelings of not being accepted by, or acceptable to, the "right" people, he used pot and cocaine to escape. He sank further into the murky abyss of depression.

The girls on the unit spotted Michael immediately. With his dark good looks and finely chiseled features, he looked like an Adonis. He knew that he was noticed, and he loved every minute of it. He played it to the hilt, as a gentleman or a cad, reminding me of the roles Cary Grant played in his old movies.

He was a bright kid, and his intelligence, coupled with his street smarts, frequently gave him an edge over the other kids. He might conceivably have become a lawyer, were it not for some serious character deficits: he lacked any realistic sense of how his actions impacted upon others or reflected back upon himself, and what was more, he didn't seem to care.

Michael and Daniel had a lot in common and very naturally gravitated toward a quick, albeit stolid, friendship. They traded war stories and played a lot of "can you top this?" They flirted with the girls. There were lots of laughs and adolescent male posturing and bravado. And very skillfully hidden beneath it all was a great deal of sadness.

One of the girls who had her eye on Michael was thirteen-year-old Kayla. Kayla didn't have many friends because, as she put it, "When the parents meet me, they don't want their kids to hang around with me. They tell 'em, 'don't bring her here no more'." She wagged her finger to make her point.

My guess was that part of it was her tattoos and multiple nose and lip piercings. Another possible contributor to her difficulty making and keeping friends was her straight-forwardness. One thing about Kayla, you always knew where you stood. You might not like it, but you always knew.

She lived, as do many kids these days, with a never-married mother, younger brother and sister. Her mother had no extended family or other support, and she described Kayla as "hostile and uncontrollable". She was at a total loss about what to do with, or for, her daughter. Kayla had run away several times and was hanging out with an older crowd. The most recent time, she was gone for ten days before the police picked her up joy riding in a stolen car with three nineteen-year-old men. One of them was a "friend"; she had never met the other two before.

Kayla didn't see anything untoward about riding around in a "borrowed" car, nor could she see any potential problem with being the only female in the company of three older males. "They're my friends," she said. "Grown ups are so stupid sometimes. Nothing would've happened."

She openly acknowledged being sexually active, and despite two pregnancy scares, she continued to be rather indiscriminate, both in her choice of sexual partners and in her behavior. She used no form of birth control and rejected the use of condoms, saying, "Guys don't like 'em." When she was admitted to Oak Haven, she had old and new "hickeys" all around her neck and upper chest.

She liked her life. "I just don't like rules," she declared. "I don't see why I have to do what somebody else tells me to do. It's *my* life."

It's my life. If I had a nickel for every time I've heard that …

At some point, my generation gave our children the notion that they are equals with adults. I'm not speaking of equality in a human rights manner, nor in any sense of their being of lesser value. I am talking about the respective roles of adult and child that have become so blurred that neither clearly understands their rights and responsibilities, nor what should be reasonably expected of each.

For many of my generation, our disillusionment with government and other established American institutions hit hard following the turbulent '60s. The call to "never trust anyone over thirty" was heard. and traditional authority was seen as untrustworthy and deceptive. We sought a new America founded on the principles of peace, love, and brotherhood coupled with "if it feels good, do it." With a goal of having fun and feeling fine, we wanted nothing to do with responsibility or what we perceived as outdated morality, achievement, and self-discipline. *My* desires became more important than *your* needs. The focus was on self rather than on society.

As we began having children, our distrust of the establishment increased. We questioned the imposition of values and discipline by others and encouraged social relevance. We challenged schools, churches, and the media to emphasize socialization over basic academic curricula. As we matured, however, we realized things weren't working. We blamed the schools. Schools blamed the home. The church blamed government. No one was willing to take responsibility or look for a way to deal with the problems.

And our children suffered.

They had no clear understanding of who had authority for what. Who's in charge? Who makes the rules? What's expected of me? What should I do? Cognitively incapable of understanding and unfamiliar with the world and its accompanying risks and responsibilities, our children tried to step forward and seize control themselves.

And still they suffer.

"It's my life," Kayla repeated, as if to make sure I was clear about what she was saying.

I liked Kayla, I genuinely liked her. Despite her oppositionality, she was spirited and her eyes sparkled when she spoke. Even though she challenged any and every adult directive, she sometimes responded to good-natured cajoling. When she wanted to. The trouble was, she believed she had all the answers and had the right to do anything and everything she wanted and to do it *her* way. So far it hadn't worked.

The Forgotten Future

*   *   *   *

During Thursday afternoon's group, the kids discussed why they were at Oak Haven. Typically, most of them were angrily indignant about being "forced into this hell hole".

In reality, Oak Haven was not exactly my idea of *Hell*. Aesthetically, the surroundings were quite pleasant, considering the not-infrequent damage done by the kids. The custodians were kept busy repairing holes in the walls, damaged paint and wallpaper, clogged toilets and broken furniture, but overall it wasn't bad. At least the walls were painted and papered, the carpeting was relatively new, and although worn, the furniture was adequate. The plastic and Plexiglas-framed pictures on the walls had to be bolted so they couldn't be removed and used as weapons, and there was even a small bookcase filled with books and board games. Like I said, not quite my idea of Hell.

Décor aside, most staff members cared very much about the kids who were entrusted to our care, and we tried to show it. There were members of the staff who brought in treats for the kids and clothing and books for those who needed them. We laughed and cried with the kids, and we worried about what would happen to them and where they would go after discharge. We tried to teach them the socially-acceptable behavior that they would need to be successful. In many cases we grew to love them.

The kids usually had a very different perspective on their stay at Oak Haven, however. For many of the kids, it was the first time rules had been invoked or enforced with any consistency, and they didn't like it. They were being asked some tough questions, and their responses and behaviors were being challenged.

There were, of course, the expected complaints about being at Oak Haven—in principle—and about other things such as the food, the sleeping arrangements, the "boredom" factor. Sometimes a teen would come in acknowledging that maybe, just *maybe*, things were getting out of hand at home and allow that perhaps some changes should be made. Usually though, those thoughts came later, if they came at all. Many times when the kids were being discharged there would be hugs and thanks and vows that their lives had been changed—and in some cases they had. But those feelings of gratitude took time to evolve. Early on, the expression of anger and hostility were pretty predictable.

Once they moved beyond the idea of being there, the kids liked to tell us how stupid the rules were. I had to admit, silently, of course, that some of the rules *were* stupid, but the rules were the rules, and the over-whelming majority of the rules were for patient safety.

Each psychiatric facility has its own *dos* and *don'ts*, *cans* and *cannots*. For example, there may be differences in who may visit patients at what point in their hospitalization. At Oak Haven, no visitors were allowed for the first twenty-four hours, after which only parents were allowed to visit. After some progress was shown on the part of the patient, brothers, sisters, and grandparents were permitted to visit, and after still more progress, friends approved by the parents could visit.

Generally, mental health institutions designate certain items as *contraband,* and these are not allowed on the unit at all. Disallowed items include sharps (glass, sharp plastic, scissors, razors, needles, nail clippers, and others), alcohol (perfume, mouthwash, and so forth), and books and magazines of a sexually-provocative or violent nature. Depending on the character of the unit and the status of individual patients, shoelaces and belts may also be taken away for safety.

Other rules that vary from facility to facility include those regarding phone calls, iPods and other radios or music players, clothing, hair bandanas, do rags, and baseball caps, jewelry and nail polish, soda and candy, and bedtimes. There are rules about patient-to-patient contact as well as staff-patient contact. Sometimes even an encouraging hug or a pat on the back is disallowed.

I broke the hugging rule a lot.

Some of the rules are for therapeutic reasons, some are for safety, and some are to give the patients something to work toward, a sort of "carrot on a stick reward" for making progress in treatment.

Just a few years ago a major source of contention in mental

health facilities was patient smoking. Hospitals, particularly psychiatric hospitals, commonly permitted even teenagers to smoke in some sort of smoking lounge. It was believed that to deprive patients of their cigarettes at such a stressful time would be unreasonable. Expecting them to give up smoking was seen as an additional and unnecessary stressor. Within adolescent units, the privilege of smoking was usually to be earned, and while the adolescents were closely monitored, they were usually allowed to continue their habit with parental permission. Newly-admitted patients who had not yet earned the privilege frequently became angry and belligerent. Often there was an epithet-scattered declaration of "I'm not staying here if I can't smoke!"

As government intervention and public intolerance of smoking grew, however, hospitals began to prohibit smoking and today most permit smoking only outside the building. At Oak Haven, we didn't allow the kids to smoke at all. Ever. Our reasons were that it was unhealthy and given their ages, illegal. Today, adolescent smokers are usually given the option of using nicotine gum or a nicotine patch to silence their cravings.

Whatever the rules, and whatever explanations the staff offer for the imposition of those rules, the teens think they are unnecessary and punitive, that they have "rights", and that they can do as they please. But that's why most of them have been hospitalized—behaving and doing exactly as they want.

Most of the rules have been put into place for valid reasons, especially those for safety. It's hard-won experience that gives staff the awareness of items that can be used by one or another of the kids to harm themselves or others, and it's the staff who are responsible for the safety of everyone on the unit. Judgment calls on disallowed items often lead to negative confrontations with patients.

As for the rules about things like baseball caps and chewing gum and certain types of magazines, there are reasons for their prohibition, too, but you won't find many staff members willing to engage in a debate over their patient's Constitutional rights as they relate to such things.

The kids think that's stupid, too.

Chapter 2
These Walls

"**H**elp! Staff! There's a fight!"

I quickly looked up from my paperwork and saw kids frantically waving their arms and motioning for us to hurry. Jackie and I both jumped up as she yelled over her shoulder to Barry, one of our new techs, "Call Dr. Strong!"

We found Daniel midway down the hall, straddling Michael, pinning him down and slamming his head into the floor. Grasping Michael's collar, he pressed his fists into Michael's throat and screamed, "I ought to kill you, you fuckin' bastard!"

I quickly stooped and pulled hard at Daniel's arms. I couldn't budge him. He was too strong; he was simply too big. I looked back over my shoulder and realized with dismay that no one had responded to our calls for assistance. My only backup was Jackie. Seven-months-pregnant Jackie.

"Jackie, get out of here! *Now!*" I barked at her, not very nicely. Then, as loudly as I could, "*We need some help down here!*"

Of all the staff I have worked with, I especially liked working with Jackie. She was a real professional. She was knowledgeable about adolescent mental health issues and had a good understanding of teen culture. She immediately responded to situations where help was needed, usually more concerned about others' safety than her own. Just like now. Except at this point in her pregnancy, this was not where she should be.

She hesitated only a moment and then backed away, turned, and ran to look for help.

It seemed to take forever. I could barely manage enough counter-pressure to keep Daniel from choking Michael, and I tried to pry Daniel's fingers loose. I silently wondered *where the hell is everybody*? Michael just lay there, gazing up at the ceiling, not struggling or fighting back. Not even moving.

Making little guttural noises.

Then, without my realizing it, Barry arrived and was standing silently beside us. He bent over at the waist, hands resting on his knees. He tried to be therapeutic, but his voice sounded like a late-night pillow talk radio host when he asked me Daniel's name. I told him, and he said softly, "Daniel, you shouldn't be doing this. If you're angry, there are other ways to handle it. Daniel ... come on now, Daniel." Barry was polite, but he certainly wasn't helping any.

Daniel kept up the pressure, and then I felt him push even harder on Michael's neck. Michael shifted slightly under the pressure, but he still didn't resist. The throaty noises continued.

Recognizing that I couldn't hold on much longer, Seth, a large and usually uninvolved kid, stepped in and grabbed Daniel under the arms and pulled him clear of Michael. As he did this, several techs from other units arrived, and a couple of them grabbed Daniel and carried him, punching and kicking and swearing, to the seclusion room.

Michael struggled to his feet and shook himself off, brushing imaginary dust from his shins and backside. He rubbed his reddened neck and insisted that he was fine, but he refused to let me check him over. He wasn't interested in talking about what had happened or how the fight had started. He mumbled, "It's okay, it was nothing," and then turned and headed toward his room.

As might be expected, though, the other kids couldn't wait to tell me about it. They thrived on excitement and so far this was the highlight of their day. The way they told it, when both boys were leaving the community room, Michael had bumped into Daniel as he passed. Whether it was intentional or not wasn't clear, but Daniel took it as overtly aggressive. He viewed it as an attack, and shoved Michael into the wall. Daniel then pushed Michael to the ground and started kicking him. The kids said Michael didn't fight back or even try to defend himself. He just lay there getting pummeled.

We listened to a few of their reports, and then Jackie and I directed the kids back to their rooms to get ready for the next group. For the time being, the excitement was over.

Once we were back in the nurses' office, however, Jackie was furious. Any time there was a violent situation like this, the normal staff response was to go in and break it up. Jackie naturally reacted the same way. Considering her very-pregnant state, however, she shouldn't be expected to get into such things and, anyway, once an alarm is sounded the expectation is that assistance will arrive quickly to help out at what can very quickly become a dangerous situation for staff and patients alike. An overhead page of "Dr. Strong!" is a call for all available hospital staff to respond *stat* to whatever area is requesting assistance.

In this case, Barry was on the unit and should have been on the scene immediately. The problem was … he wasn't. Jackie said he didn't even move. He just stood in the nurses' office, immobile, gazing down the hall. Like a deer caught in the headlights. His response to Jackie's, "*You have to get down there and help Debbi*!" was a fainthearted, "But I haven't taken the violence management class yet …"

Only after Jackie's insistent, "*Godammit Barry*! I don't care what you've taken or what you haven't taken! Get down there and help!" had Barry moved to my side and began to speak oh-so-softly and futilely to Daniel.

I glanced over at Barry, who was standing a few feet away and who was taking this all in while trying to appear otherwise occupied. He was new to the psy-world, but everyone who works in such surroundings needs to be able to think on his feet. Quickly and without hesitation. The strange, new terrain of a locked psychiatric unit can be terrifying to anyone who is unfamiliar with it, and stereotypes about mental health patients abound. While I could understand his reluctance to get involved without proper training, he should never have been working on the unit until he was prepared, for our benefit as well as that of the patients.

Unfortunately, violence management classes, which include various techniques of verbal de-escalation as a way to safely calm patients before more aggressive measures are necessary, were held only twice a year, and another wouldn't be scheduled for several months. The hospital administration liked to have a full class when they did the training since they felt it wasn't cost-effective to teach only three or four.

Incidents like this were early indicators that the hospital administration's growing concern over cost-containment and numbers of staff—what are known as FTEs (full time equivalents)—coupled with managed care's growing omnipotence, would more and more often mean inadequate backup for violent situations as well as less than optimal staffing to adequately meet the needs of our patients. And unfortunately, at a much later time, some of us would learn that much of the training we did receive was inadequate in many areas and in many ways.

* * * *

When I returned to the unit after my weekend off, the halls were empty. No noise. No kids in sight.

Naturally, I was curious as I entered the nurses' office. A few seconds later Robin, the day shift nurse, arrived and dropped the day board loudly on the desk.

"I am *so* glad you're here," she said, not looking particularly happy. "This has been a really rough day."

"Oh yeah? Well, I'm glad to see you, too, Robin. Did all the kids go home?" I joked as I peered through the safety glass window which looked out over the length of the hall.

"Room restriction," Robin said simply. "I'll tell you in report, but the gist is that some of the girls pierced their noses last night, so everybody's on room restriction." She picked up the Kardex and day board, and I followed her down the hall. "*Let's go! I want to go home.*"

The Forgotten Future

I learned during report that the kids had been so taken with Kayla's nose rings that four girls had self-pierced their noses on Sunday night. When they came out for breakfast Monday morning, their angry-looking, red noses had small studs in place.

As it turned out, almost all the kids knew of their plans before the fact. As might be expected, though, no one saw any reason to let staff know about it, probably because they all knew staff would never permit it.

Everyone was placed on room restriction until 10:00 Monday night; by then they would be—should be—in bed. The kids thought the room restriction was an overreaction, but the policy for something like this demanded consequences for the entire unit. The kids, once again, didn't understand why staff interfered in their business or why we cared whether or not they had pierced their noses

No decision had yet been made regarding further consequences for the piercings, but possibilities such as banning earrings or even all jewelry were being considered by those higher up. The parents of those kids who now had holes in their noses where none had been before had been notified, but I couldn't imagine they had received it as good news.

Meanwhile, when I made my rounds, I was sure to take along plenty of alcohol pledgets to keep their red noses from becoming infected.

* * * *

Room restriction for the entire unit didn't happen often. When it did, I usually enjoyed it, but not for reasons others might suspect.

With kids on room restriction, we were freed from putting out fires; that is, breaking up small altercations or disagreements, watching and monitoring males and females lest their therapeutic alliances get out of hand, and moving kids from room-to-room and group-to-group. It afforded us an opportunity to actually spend time talking one-to-one with kids without outside distractions, to find out how they were doing, what they were thinking and feeling, what they wanted to change, what they feared, and what they dreamed. It was an opportunity to get to know the kids and for them to get to know us. As people. Not as adults or as their keepers, but as people who cared about them.

People like to talk about the new openness between kids and their parents, an openness that allows two generations to calmly and lovingly explore and discuss such formidable issues as sex, birth control, substance abuse, hopes, and dreams.

These same people speak of an openness that allows young people to express their thoughts and feelings to the adults in their lives without fear of a negative response or reprisal. Freedom of speech, in homes where parent and child are friends.

This may be true in some homes: the homes of policy makers, the homes with sensitive and caring parents, the homes of those families who value their children just because they *are*. Unfortunately, there are an untold number of homes in which asking a question about sexuality carries with it the risk of being called a slut or a 'ho. Homes in which discussion about substance abuse takes place as parent and child get high together. Homes in which a child who voices an opinion is invited to "shut up or leave". Homes in which sex education includes a father sleeping with his daughter.

It's hard for kids from such homes to trust anyone enough to tell them about their lives, their feelings, or their experiences. They fear being shamed or rejected or ridiculed, and it takes courage to open up and risk being hurt. Again.

But on the unit, in those times filled with stillness, the kids can feel a caring that reaches beyond the walls they have erected. Those times can be an interlude that sustains and nourishes the hearts of the young and carries them forward. And, sometimes, those times can help a tired nurse or doctor or mental health tech feel that maybe, just maybe, he or she can make a difference.

* * * *

As dedicated to helping and as desirous of facilitating positive growth in our patients as the employees of Oak Haven and other such facilities are, a unit staffed with three—or even four—people for twelve to fifteen or sixteen teenagers or more can be hectic even under the best of circumstances. Most child and adolescent units have only one registered nurse on the unit at any given time. It is the nurse's responsibility to do assessments, write and update care plans, pour and pass medications, monitor patients' mental and physical status, do staffing assignments, speak with physicians and accept physician's orders, do one-to-ones with patients, monitor any takedowns and/or restraints, do the preponderance of each shift's charting, complete patient admissions and discharges, and a myriad of other tasks. The worst staffing conditions under which I have worked was being the only nurse on a unit with four MHTs and thirty-one patients between the ages of three and twelve. That's right. One nurse carrying for for 31 patients under the age of twelve.

With the nurse occupied with the "professional" tasks that only she can do, the job of "policing", i.e., monitoring the unit in its entirety, falls on the shoulders of the MHTs, who may or may not even hold a two-year college degree. Attempting to provide anything particularly therapeutic with such staffing is impossible, and sometimes it comes down to feeling that a successful shift is one in which no one is hurt.

Oak Haven's staffing guidelines called for one staff person for every five adolescents, and this is typical for inpatient adolescent mental health units. This guideline was, of course, stretched a little as in *ten kids need two staff ... and eleven is just one more than ten ... and twelve is just one more than that ...* and so on. Although the hospital's administration did a lot of nodding and *yes-ing* and providing assurances that our concerns regarding the acuity—i.e., the types of disorders and their severity, the intensity in which those disorders' symptoms and behaviors are expressed, and the level and types of care needed to adequately meet the patients' needs—of the unit were being considered, when it came right down to dollars and cents vs. calling in additional staff, it really didn't make much difference whether we had a unit full of despondent adolescents or a unit full of destructively conduct-disordered kids. The staff-to-patient ratio stayed pretty much the same, despite the different types of treatment and management required by each patient.

Deborah Clark Ebel, R.N.

Staffing costs are the lion's share of a hospital's expenses and, unfortunately, if hospital costs continue to escalate, many people and insurances will find affordable mental health care impossible to find. At the same time, responsible people must rightly question the ability of inpatient psychiatric facilities to address competently and adequately the needs of increasing numbers of children and adolescents. One must ask how much do most of the hospitalized young people actually benefit from short-term hospitalization, given short-staffing ratios and severely curtailed services? What methods and new modalities might be developed to properly and more effectively provide for such a fast-growing population of children who are in need of services and deserve the best that we can offer?

*   *   *   *

"I ain't fuckin' talkin' to nobody!" Daniel was furious. He had just learned during a family therapy session that his mother was refusing to allow him to return home. Despite Daniel's promises to forswear forever all alcohol and drugs, both Margie, the unit social worker, and Daniel's mother felt he should spend some time in a drug rehab following discharge from Oak Haven. Dr. Evans, away at a medical conference, had already discussed placement with Margie and was in full agreement.

"Just stay the fuck away from me," Daniel growled as he walked into his room and punched the closet door. Margie stood in the doorway talking softly to him for a few minutes, then came to the nurses' office.

"He's okay. He's upset about not going home ..." she sighed. "He just doesn't understand that even with all his promises, unless he gets additional clean time before going home, he's going to pick up and use again." She shook her head and repeated, "He just doesn't get it. He still thinks he can go home and hang out with his old friends and just say 'no'."

"Yeah, right. And then he'll be right back where he was when he came in here," agreed Howard.

Howard was one of our MHTs. He was also one of the best

things to happen at Oak Haven in a long time. For far too long the presence of male nurses or male techs was only a once-in-a-while occurrence, and it is only recently that males have become commonplace figures. It isn't that women are incapable of handling situations as they arise; rather, the benefit of a male staff presence is two-fold.

A lot of our kids had never had any positive adult male role models in their lives, and it was important that they see men responsibly engaged in serious activities. The only contact many of our kids had ever had with adult males was in abusive relationships of one type or another. That, and the police.

Young men can gain much from exchanging thoughts and feelings with male staff, and the male staff could frequently offer perspectives very different from those of a female simply because they had spent their youth as teenage boys. The kids needed men they could look up to, men they could respect and who respected them back.

Secondly and very pragmatically, the appearance of a large, no-nonsense, male in the midst of a high-pressure situation could often keep things from deteriorating further. An angry kid who wouldn't hesitate to barrel right over a female might think twice before charging a male.

Howard fit the bill perfectly: a down-to-earth guy who pulled no punches, yet was sensitive and genuine in his desire to work with the kids.

A no-bullshit kind of guy.

*　　*　　*　　*

Since his fight with Daniel, Michael had become markedly quieter and more introspective. He continued to be the braggadocio among his peers, but whenever he thought no one was looking, his extreme sadness was evident. He still refused to discuss his fight with Daniel, and we remained mystified over his complete and total unwillingness to defend himself when he was attacked.

That Monday, Michael meandered into the community room for the final group of the evening, *Wrap Up*. Wrap Up wasn't in-

Deborah Clark Ebel, R.N.

tended to be formal group therapy, but rather a time to look back at the day's events and think about what went wrong, what went right, what each person might have said or done differently, and get a head start on planning for the next day. It was a way to give what is referred to as *closure* to the day. The idea was for everyone in the group to have some time to wind down and find some peace, although it didn't always work out that way.

We bowed our heads and began with the Serenity Prayer:

God,
grant me the serenity to accept the things I cannot change,
the courage to change the things I can, and
the wisdom to know the difference.

Every morning, each patient set a goal to be accomplished that day. It had to be treatment-focused, specific, and measurable. A patient who was withdrawn and tended to isolate in his room might set a goal to spend all his free time in the community room with peers. Another might have the goal of disclosing her drug use to her parents. Still another might try to avoid being verbally or physically abusive toward peers and staff.

Wrap Up was a time when the kids could talk freely about whether or not they had accomplished their goals, why or why not, and anything else on their minds.

Dea offered to begin, and she spoke of her goal to control her anger when her mother and brother visited. She and her brother could be an explosive combination, and it seemed that they often did things to deliberately set each other off. This evening's visit was the first time she had seen her brother since her admission to Oak Haven, and she had been pretty anxious earlier in the day. Shortly before coming to Oak Haven, she had sold her brother's bike and he had, understandably, been more than a little upset. We all wondered how things had gone during their visit.

"It went okay," she said confidently. "We worked things out. I don't even have to pay him back 'cause my mom says I was crazy when I came to Oak Haven." She raised her eyebrows and smirked, "Now, I'm not crazy no more." She knew she was getting

~ 36 ~

away with something she shouldn't.

Kayla hugged her knees to her chest and rocked back and forth. "So, why'd you sell his bike, anyways?"

"Cause mine got stole, and I didn't want him to have one if I didn't." Her nebulous logic sounded almost righteous. "That wouldn't be fair." Dea nodded, indicating that as far as she was concerned, the matter was closed.

"Dea, what does your brother think of this?" I had to ask, since my understanding of *fair* was obviously different from hers.

"Oh, he don't mind. My mom is buyin' him and me both new bikes." Her singsong reply told me she didn't quite get the point, but that she didn't really care, either.

Kayla was next. Her goal had been to call her mom. She hadn't heard from her mother since her pass a week ago, and she was still unable to reach her today. "She's busy, y'know, with getting ready for the move and everything."

Before Kayla came to the hospital, her mom had been talking about moving several hundred miles away, but whether or not the move would actually take place hadn't yet been decided. In any event, her mom hadn't called, even though she didn't have a job to take up her time. Her family, like many others, collected welfare benefits and the hospital costs were covered by government assistance.

"I can try again tomorrow, and anyway, on the weekend, she'll prob'ly come see me. Prob'ly." She nodded as a way of reassuring herself, but I didn't think she really believed what she was saying. A lot of our kids never received visitors during their entire stay at the hospital. Tragically, for a lot of our kids, it was out of sight, out of mind.

I hoped that wouldn't be the case with Kayla.

Now, it was Michael's turn. Two years before, his twin had been killed when the car their mother was driving spun out of control and went over an embankment. There were rumors that she had been drinking, but no charges were ever brought against her. Michael's goal today was to talk about his brother, something he had avoided since the accident.

Now he hesitated, playing with his shoelace. Then, "I have to tell you about my brother." His voice was thick.

We waited thirty seconds or so, but it seemed like much longer. Michael took a deep breath and began what must have taken an enormous amount of courage. "Matt was my best friend. He was my brother, but he was more than a brother, y'know? I was three minutes older, and I always used to kid him about being my little brother." He paused at what should have been a fond memory, but wasn't. He twisted his shoelace around his finger.

"He was really smart and really good." Tears welled up and spilled over onto his cheeks. "He came to visit me when I was at Whittimore House for drugs. My mom brought him and we were supposed to go out on a pass. I got really pissed when I saw Matt 'cause he was wearin' one of my best shirts. I hated it when he took my clothes." He swallowed hard and wiped tears from his cheeks with the backs of his hands. He pressed his fists into his eyes as if trying to push back a memory.

The rest of the kids were silent, some biting their lips, some hugging their legs to their chests, some looking straight at Michael, and some unable to look at anything except their laps or the floor where they sat. They identified with Michael being in pain, but they weren't quite sure where this was going.

"I yelled and he yelled and we both got more and more pissed 'til my mom finally said, 'Forget it! I'm not taking the two of you anywhere!' and they were gonna leave. I was really ripshit y'know, 'cause first he was wearin' my clothes while I was in that fuckin' place, and now I couldn't even go out on pass."

He looked at us for the first time, his face red and damp. "I told him I hated him and I had always hated him and I wished he was dead. And he died. They crashed on the way home." He made a choking, convulsive sound and gasped, "It shoulda been me. Oh, God ... it shoulda been me!"

He wasn't looking at us anymore. He was lost in his own pain. What he wanted was something we couldn't give him: his brother's forgiveness. What he needed was to forgive himself.

The group was silent, allowing the impact of what we had just heard sink in. My throat was tight and my mind raced. I looked at the boy sitting across from me and thought of the heavy burden he carried. How do you ever get out from under something like that?

His final words to the brother he loved: *I wish you were dead.* We watched as Michael buried his face in his folded arms and was engulfed by disconsolate, body-wracking sobs.

After lights out, I thought a lot about Michael and Matt, about how everyone gets mad sometimes and says things they don't mean. At best the exchange is forgiven, if not forgotten, and people continue on with the relationship. Perhaps the worst that might happen is the relationship is irrevocably damaged. Maybe it even ends. In Michael's case, though, he would forever carry the knowledge that the last words he ever spoke to his brother were a wish for his death.

And as if losing his twin were not punishment enough, he was now playing their parting over and over in his mind. He could never change what happened, but the question was *could he learn to grow beyond the tragedy that was haunting him*?

*   *   *   *

I arrived at work several days later to find that there had been problems during the night. Big problems. The kids were in a group off the unit when Robin began report with a tightly clinched jaw. "You have seventeen patients. Daniel was transferred to Longmeadow today." She drew in a deep breath and continued slowly, "Daniel tried to hang himself last night in the closet. Cleo found him in the same room as that other guy."

"Oh, no!" The news about Daniel was bad enough, but knowing that Cleo was the one who had found him made things even worse. "Is he all right? Was he unconscious? What about Cleo? How is she?"

Cleo was the 11 p.m. to 7:30 a.m. night shift nurse, a kind and caring nurse who appreciated the quiet afforded by the night shift. A year or so earlier she had discovered the body of a patient from the adult unit who had wandered into an empty room on the adolescent unit and hanged himself. When the adult unit staff had been unable to find him, an alert was sent out to adjacent units. Cleo had responded by checking all our rooms and bathrooms and discovered him hanging from the shower rod. Dead.

I can imagine few things more upsetting professionally than to have a patient for whom I am responsible take his own life. Cleo struggled with that for a long time before she reconciled herself that there was nothing she could have done differently given the same set of circumstances.

Shortly after that patient's death, it was ordered that all the units' shower and closet rods be replaced with breakaway rods designed to collapse under a minimum weight. Obviously they hadn't all been changed, and I didn't understand why, if they were not replaced, why they were not simply removed. In any case they hadn't been, and now we had another hanging.

Oak Haven's medical director quickly made the decision to transfer Daniel to Longmeadow Behavioral Healthcare, and Daniel was moved by transport ambulance shortly before noon. Longmeadow had a corporate affiliation with Oak Haven and had a larger and better-staffed close observation unit that could provide a more secure environment for those who were acutely suicidal.

"Cleo gave me the shift report this morning, and she was really shaken up. The kids were upset when they found out about Daniel, especially Michael," continued Robin, sounding tense. "He went into his room and started punching the wall, so we had to safety coat him for a while. I think he's okay now, but keep an eye on him."

After report I walked into Daniel's now-empty room, opened the closet door and reached up and grabbed the rod. I gave a few tugs, tentative at first, then more demanding, with weight and force. Nothing. It held. Handy for holding heavy clothing; not so helpful for holding hanging people.

I rested my head on my outstretched arm and tried to imagine how alone Daniel must have felt when he climbed into the closet, intending to die. I closed my eyes and wondered about the transition some take from infant to child to teenager to teenager-so-distraught-that-life-has-only-one-meaning: more pain. When does the hurt and neglect begin to take its toll? When does one stop growing and begin deteriorating?

Daniel was not the first teenager to try to end his life, and he would not be the last. There was something especially tragic, though, about his view of death as the only way out in a place where he should have felt protected and safe.

Checking my watch I realized the kids would be returning from their group. I made a mental note to call Cleo later and shut the closet door tight.

In 2007, the American Academy of Child and Adolescent Psychiatry (AACAP) issued a special press release concerning the alarming increase in the suicide rate for young people ages one to nineteen: an 18.2 percent increase from 2003 to 2004. Suicide is the third leading cause of death in the United States for fifteen to twenty-year-olds and the sixth leading cause of death for five to fourteen-year-olds. Approximately two million adolescents attempt suicide each year, and almost 700,000 require medical attention for their attempt. And, unfortunately, the rate of death by suicide may actually be higher than reported because some of these deaths may have been incorrectly labeled "accidents".

This time, Daniel wasn't successful in ending his life. *This time* ...

*   *   *   *

Kids can be extraordinarily cruel to each other sometimes. They pick up on another's perceived vulnerability and hammer away until they get the response they're after—embarrassment, humiliation, anger, shame—whatever.

I've never understood what it is within some people that drives them to deliberately hurt another, and I understand it even less within the hospital setting. Everyone in a psychiatric hospital is in some state of discomfort or turmoil, but some patients choose to inflict additional pain on their peers instead of bonding with them. Maybe it's their way of getting even with a world they feel has given them a raw deal.

Seth was a kind and gentle sixteen-year-old who weighed-in at close to three hundred pounds and who had been admitted with major depression. He also had a congenital speech impediment. He'd been made to feel inferior, both at home and at school, and he usually tried to stay out of everyone's way to avoid any more negative experiences. When he first arrived at Oak Haven, he rarely made eye contact with anyone, never spoke in groups, and didn't interact with the other kids unless he absolutely had to.

Through hard work on his part, he had gradually started to try new things. To stretch and dare to risk things he had never allowed himself to do before. He was conscientious and wanted so much to grow and change that he eventually became the senior member of the community. For the first time in his life, he felt proud of his accomplishments. One of his new responsibilities was running the evening community meetings.

During Seth's third evening as community chairperson, Dea angrily confronted Meghan about what she perceived as Meghan's negative attitude and verbal abuse of a couple of their peers. As things grew louder and more intense, and as difficult as it was, Seth intervened, trying to mediate what was happening.

Dea turned on him with venom. "Why can't you talk so people can understand you? *You go' 'uh uh uh duh duh duh* ... You sound like you got a mouth full of shit. You *look* like you got a big fat mouth full of shit! Shitmouth ..."

Seth paled, like he had been slapped. A couple of kids giggled.

I waited to see where things would go, whether Seth could handle it, whether someone else in the group would call Dea on her nastiness.

No one said a word.

"I, uh, I ... tink ..." Seth was lost.

Silence.

My gut reaction was that I wanted to attack Dea for her rudeness, that I wanted to point out that she was doing exactly what she had accused Meghan of doing and that she was attacking someone who was likely to be damaged by her anger. I wanted to tell her how angry and disappointed I was. But that wouldn't have accomplished anything and, besides, that's probably what she expected from staff.

My job was to help teach and model behavior, even when I didn't feel like it, and so I spoke calmly and deliberately. "Dea, sometimes some people are harder to understand than others. It might be because they have an accent, or the community where they were raised uses a lot of what are called colloquialisms, or in some cases because there is some sort of a physical problem with their speech. I think everyone here knows Seth has had surgery for his speech …"

I looked around the room before settling my gaze on Dea.

"I think Seth has done a fine job running the community meetings so far. Right now I think he was just trying to help clear things up between you and Meghan."

Absolute silence.

Dea's eyes flashed. "If he's gonna talk to me … man, he better learn how to speak." She looked at Seth with hatred. "God, man, nobody can understand a fuckin' thing you say."

I gave her a sharp look and then tried to get the meeting back on track. There wasn't any use in trying to further reason with Dea because she just didn't get it. Seth didn't speak again during the meeting, which didn't surprise me.

We got through the rest of the meeting somehow, but afterward Seth approached me in the hall.

"I … I … I … do'n tink I can run no more meetins'," he said sadly. His eyes were moist. "It's jus' too mush. They can't unnerstan' me … I jus' feld myself so *pissed*, like I wanten' to get up and smash her or somethin'."

Or, I suspected, like he wanted to smash himself or something. Then, he turned and walked away, down the hall, muttering to himself.

*   *   *   *

When Michael was admitted, we found that he had been refusing to take his lithium for several months. He had now been taking it in the hospital for three weeks and was beginning to show some positive effects of the medication. His weekly blood test showed the level of the drug in his bloodstream to be within what is referred to as the *therapeutic range*, meaning there is enough (yet not so much that it might harm him) medication in his body to be of benefit.

Michael's willingness to begin to talk about his final meeting with his brother was quite significant, and we hoped he could now start to work on his unresolved grief. That is, if he chose to. Ultimately, the choice was up to him, whether he decided to work it through and move on or continue to run from his past and bury his pain in drugs and avoidance.

In any event, Dr. Evans planned to discharge Michael back home in a few days, and Michael's mom had already enrolled him in the community alternative high school.

We had noticed, though, that since the other kids had learned about his brother's death during Wrap Up, the girls had taken to being his caretakers. While it was good and positive that he had shared his grief with the group, we were concerned about the amount of secondary gain he was getting from his revelation. In other words, how much mileage was he getting out of the situation? What were the benefits of his display of sorrow and sadness?

The fine line to be walked in a situation like this was that while it was important that Michael acknowledge the events surrounding his brother's death, too much sympathetic attention might actually prevent him from dealing with the matter and moving on. He had already begun to retreat back into his *machismo* image, the image that said "nothing touches me, nothing hurts me".

We were concerned that too much focus on Michael by his peers would keep them from working on their own issues. What could be—and most certainly would be—construed by the other patients as a grieving young man receiving comfort from friends was in reality an opportunity for the others to avoid having to deal with their own problems.

While Kayla appeared to have lost interest in Michael, fourteen-year-old Rachel had taken to following him around on a self-assigned invisible leash. She seemed to see it as her personal mission to carry Michael's point card, get extra milk for his meals from the kitchen, and jump in to rescue him—because she "understood" him, and "staff" didn't—should he be put on the spot. Michael didn't seem to be actively encouraging her attention and assistance, but he was certainly reveling in it.

As the evening wore on and I had a chance to speak with some of the kids, I reflected on how easy it is to replace, at least on the surface, sadness over things like death with indignation over petty squabbles. Suicide was painful to contemplate; it was much easier to get angry over who sat where during movie time.

*   *   *   *

I opened the door to Vickie's room and found her in bed with the lights on. She quickly grabbed the covers and pulled them chest high. "Oh! You scared me!"

Was it my imagination or did she have GUILT written in flashing neon colors all over her face? "What are you doing, Vickie? It's almost eleven. Lights-out was a long time ago." I stood at the end of her bed.

"Nothin'. I couldn't get to sleep."

"Oh, yeah? What else?" It was a combination of instinct and frank suspicion, but things on the unit were rarely as they seemed. Besides, her haste in pulling up the blanket didn't exactly strike me as an attempt at modesty. "Can I see your arms?"

She stared at me and then asked, "Why?"

Sly.

"Because I want to see your arms."

"Why?"

"Because I do." I thought back to my mistake many years before when I first started working in mental health. I had heard a rumor about a girl cutting herself and I confronted her in a situation very similar to this. I asked to see her wrists, she complied, and both wrists were fine. I left the room.

I discovered later that I should have looked at her entire arm, not just her wrists. Her entire left upper arm was sliced to bits, with vertical and horizontal lines that looked like bloody graph paper. Since then I left nothing to chance.

"Vickie, I need to see your arms," I repeated.

She groaned and pulled both arms out from under the covers.

Clean as a whistle. Both sides. Upper arms, too. Still, I didn't feel right about things. Just one of those niggling little feelings that I couldn't quite put my finger on, but which wouldn't go away.

"Vickie, would you get out of bed for a minute. Please."

"This is stupid! I just want to go to sleep, and you fuckin' won't let me." She slammed her arms down hard on the bed and didn't make any move to get up. Defensiveness always made me even more suspicious.

"Vickie, please get out of bed. Now. Or …"

She started to climb out of bed, and even though she tried to roll the covers under so I wouldn't see, I noticed several droplets of fresh blood on the upper sheet. "Vickie …" I began.

"What? What? So what?" She twirled around with her right hand on her abdomen.

Vickie didn't have a history of self-mutilation, but my guess was that she had been cutting on her belly. It's a fairly common area the kids use because it's not readily seen.

I was wrong.

Using an earring stud, she had pierced her belly button. There was blood, a pretty fair amount.

"Vickie, I can't believe you did this after all the problems we had before with the nose rings." I held out my hand. "I need the stud."

"I need it! If I take it out, the hole will close up!"

"Too bad. I want the stud." My hand was out, but it was still empty.

"I hate this place, and I hate you! You're always tellin' us what to do. You're a fuckin bitch, and I don't know why you even work here. You must hate kids!" She threw the stud at the wall and it took me a little over five minutes to find it.

I walked back to the nurses' office, all the while thinking about how I knew she was wrong. A person really had to care about kids to work in a place like this.

*   *   *   *

Robin started report the next day. "Just to let you know, Stephen's been really pissy all day. Barry worked with us on days and told Stephen to get out of bed half a dozen times. Finally, Barry got a cup of cold water and dumped it right on top of Stephen. Stephen got up, but he's been a wild man ever since."

The Forgotten Future

She shifted her papers, "Moving right along … rooms 401A and B are empty. 402A is Meghan R. I think you admitted her a few evenings ago. Her doctor is Dr. Carmichael, and her diagnoses are polysubstance abuse and conduct disorder. She's had a bad day, needed lots of reminders about personal space. She was in Stacey's face a lot and was swearing at Dea earlier because she wouldn't move and let Meghan sit where she wanted in group therapy. She's real aggressive at times."

"Did we get any more information from Dr. Carmichael about her? He said he was going to try to get the history dictated." I hoped we had something, because it would help us understand her problems.

"Yeah, he did. I think it's …" Robin rifled through the papers on her clipboard. "Wait, I have it right here. Okay, a couple of months ago Meghan ran away from her grandmother's house and went to live with this guy, Evan. There were several other people living there, too. Evan's twenty and he's a dealer—marijuana, cocaine, and heroin. Meghan started selling for him; Dr. Carmichael says her specialty was heroin. She says she never used heroin, but she does admit to using pot and cocaine."

"Great. She's fifteen, and he's twenty, and she's selling drugs for him. Why do these girls do this?" It was strictly a rhetorical question, but I felt I had to ask it just the same.

"Who knows? Anyway all these people were dropping into and out of Evan's apartment all the time. Sometimes there were as many as twelve people staying there. In three rooms. This guy, Dirk, came on to Meghan, she liked him, and they started sleeping together."

"If the punch line is that she's pregnant, I'm quitting right now. I mean it. I'm walking right out of here."

"No, she's not pregnant, we got the lab report back on that. But that's the only good news. Dirk beat her, verbally abused her, and they had sex several times. That's statutory rape, but I don't know if there will be any charges against him. But then she says she *loves* him, so she thinks everything's okay."

Robin continued, "Basically, Dirk was a jerk. I guess he was okay when he was sober, but when he got drunk or high he would terrorize anybody who happened to be around. Dr. Carmichael says that Dirk always carried a gun—loaded—and he had a reputation for shooting at people with little provocation. Anyway, a week or so ago, Dirk walked up to Meghan when she was in the kitchen and held a gun to her forehead. Right between her eyes."

I listened, knowing, but not wanting to believe, that this kind of thing goes on every day all around us and for the most part society refuses to acknowledge it. People get angry or upset over things that are so insignificant in comparison, and then they are shocked and outraged when something is horrible enough to make the evening news. But, this was a fifteen-year-old girl we were talking about, living with and being abused by drug dealers and no one knew or cared. And she wasn't the only one.

"Okay, it says here, 'He didn't say anything. Meghan didn't move.' Dr. Carmichael says here, quote, 'They stood there, frozen, for some time, and he snapped the trigger on the gun which did not fire. He laughed and then walked out of the kitchen and through the apartment and drove away in his car. Meghan started to cry and recalls she was still sobbing several hours later when evening arrived. She still doesn't know whether Dirk intended to kill her or just scare her. Maybe he would have been satisfied with either outcome.' Unquote." Robin looked up from the report sheet and our eyes met and locked. We both knew what the other was thinking, what the other was feeling. And there was nothing to say. Nothing at all.

* * * *

Joe made animal noises. Loud ones. Sometimes unidentifiable ones. But he was funny and delightfully friendly, and sometimes he would just about break us up.

He was a really neat kid, once you got to know him. He had no social skills to speak of, his personal hygiene was terrible, and he could be abrasive and intrusive. When I first met him, he sort of reminded me of the proverbial kid reared by a pack of wolves.

Actually, that wasn't too far off.

Joe had been raised by his drug-abusing mother and had moved more than two dozen times in his fourteen years. He was a tense and difficult child who would have been a challenge even for the best parents. Unfortunately, his mother was also tense and difficult and didn't have any idea how to handle him. Sometimes she locked him in a closet. Sometimes she didn't feed him. Sometimes she didn't even speak to him for days.

When he was admitted, it was obvious that he was somewhat delayed in a number of areas and it was supposed he had below normal intelligence. We anxiously awaited the psychologist's report, and when it arrived we eagerly perused it and were surprised to learn that the psych testing showed slightly *above* normal intelligence. At the same time, we were gravely disappointed to learn how it was believed he had suffered severe developmental delays.

Apparently he had been so emotionally deprived as a youngster that he had never been able to develop normally. Verbally, socially, behaviorally—he was functioning well below his potential. Had he been raised differently, in a nurturing and caring environment, his functioning, his life, he himself, might have flourished.

Despite his emotional outbursts and frequently outrageous behavior, there was something about Joe that you couldn't help but like. He thrived under the attention he received from the staff. He enjoyed playing board games and liked to teach us card tricks. His months-long stay with us came at a time when the census was low enough that the staff actually had time to sit and play games with him. We played UNO and Monopoly, mostly.

Desperate for attention and longing for companionship, he often kept a game of Monopoly going long past winning. He excitedly gave Monopoly money to his opponents just to keep them in the game, and at the end of each game he would let out a gigantic, noisy, animal sound that sounded sort of like a combination of a belching pig and a yelping hippopotamus.

He said he never wanted to leave us because, "These walls hold me together."

A small tarnished stud adorned his left ear, and throughout his stay he repeated over and over that he hoped to get an earring with a small cross on it. *Someday.*

We gave him a small going-away party on the day of his discharge, complete with doughnuts and caffeine-free soda, and several of the staff brought in gifts. There was an Oak Haven Hospital tee shirt and mug, a cassette tape, an UNO game. As he was leaving I hugged him and slipped a small package into his hand. In it was a special earring with a cross.

I wish I could have given him more.

Chapter 3
Ice Cream

The nurses' office was crowded when Dr. Evans looked up from his charting to address anyone within earshot. "Say, did you hear about that body they pulled out of the river?" A few heads turned to listen.

"No! What happened? When?"

Evans' furrowed brow showed concern. "Well, it was a woman, and they think she was probably a nurse ..."

Now he had everyone's attention.

The river was just a short walk from Oak Haven ... My mind raced. Was it a nurse? Had she been murdered? How? Why? And who would do such a thing? We all knew there was a calculated risk of injury at work, and disturbed patients sometimes made threats ... Could her attacker be a former patient? The thought of one of one of our own actually being assaulted, even killed. It made me shudder.

Still, we all read the newspapers and watched cable news, and last year one of the male techs had gone out after work one night and found his car smeared with feces.

"Yeah, well," Evans chuckled, "they figured she was a nurse because her stomach was empty, her bladder was full, her fingers were worked to the bone, and her ass was chewed off."

He had us.

Jackie took a swat at his head as she walked past. "You're a jerk, you know that?"

He howled.

*   *   *   *

Humor is an important and necessary part of enabling staff to get through each eight-hour shift. Without it and the ability to laugh at life's incongruities, it would be difficult, if not impossible, to function within the highly-intense and emotionally-charged environment of a psychiatric unit. Such profound and unrelenting intimate contact with people in crisis can be difficult to handle for even the most dedicated and caring individuals.

The experience and expression of humor can be as simple and as open as the ability to laugh at oneself, as when a mischievous twelve-year-old greeted me with a handshake in the cafeteria. A handshake in which he held orange-flavored gelatin ... and squeezed my hand. It squished and gooshed and I squeezed back. I don't know which of us laughed harder.

Life's oddities and inconsistencies can also be reflected through the use of "dark" or "gallows" humor. Television's M*A*S*H exposed us to such humor when the overworked and war-weary surgeons told jokes and made sport of the war, their patients, and themselves in an attempt to avoid being consumed by their situation. In no instance did their use of humor give the message that war was fun or that combat was not a deadly-serious affair. On the contrary. The irony inherent in their words and in their daily lives allowed viewers to experience and acknowledge the horrors of war and the toll taken on humanity. Many times it's a matter of laughing to keep from crying. Or sometimes doing both at the same time.

Similarly, humor can be helpful to those working in the mental health field when used to release some of the pressure under which we work. Its use isn't in any way intended as a put-down or negative cut at our patients or their situations.

The feeling of empathy and a desire to help those whose lives are in turmoil are common characteristics of health care providers

The Forgotten Future

and social services professionals. The burden of being privy to the deepest, darkest, and most horrendous of thoughts, fears, feelings, and experiences is heavy.

Transitioning from the pain and despair of the psychiatric setting to the safety and comfort of our personal lives can be difficult. Our jobs are not the kind where we can walk out and turn off any conscious thought of those in our care. They are people, just like you and me, who struggle with life. They are people about whom we think and pray and cry and about whom we care, often very deeply. And it's precisely because we care so very much that we need humor to make the unbearable, bearable, and to try to make sense out of a situation that doesn't.

* * * *

I arrived at work one evening to find Cleo's locker emptied out. I wasn't surprised, but I was sad.

I saw Connie later and asked if Cleo had resigned.

"Yeah, she came in this morning to pick up her things. She said things here are just too hard to deal with, and her heart just isn't in it any more." Connie was the unit nurse manager, and she looked genuinely saddened to see Cleo go.

I didn't know what to say, other than that I was sorry. When I had spoken with Cleo shortly after Daniel's suicide attempt, she hadn't sounded well at all. She told me that the pain of working on the unit was really getting to her, and she thought perhaps she should try something new career-wise.

Things sometimes just become more than a person can bear, and no matter how much someone cares and wants to help others, there are limits to what a person can take and still maintain a balance. It's hard to see kids in pain day after day, and it's equally as challenging to cope with the verbal abuse and stress that we, as staff, faced. I could understand her calling it quits, but we would all miss her, and it was a loss to everyone.

* * * *

Deborah Clark Ebel, R.N.

It was time for group, and I was only ten minutes late … which made me just about on time. Four or five kids clamored at the nurses' office door demanding to know what was scheduled next.

I turned and said, "Look, guys. We have sexuality group in the resource room. You all know that without asking me. Just look at your schedules, and if you'll give me sixty seconds to get my stuff together, I'll meet you in there, and we'll get started."

My request was met with assorted comments like, "All *right!*" and "Yeah! Yeah! Let's have sex," snorted in a *Beavis and Butt-head* voice, and from Robert, "I don't need to go. I know all that stuff already."

I brushed my hair back out of my eyes thinking *I need a hair-cut* and looked at Jackie. "So, what do you want to do tonight?"

When we had first started doing sexuality group, we were al-ways prepared. We had time to discuss topics and plan activities in advance. These days, that was a luxury we didn't have. With staff shortages, if we actually had time to do the group at all, we felt it was a success. Then we also had to chart individually on all par-ticipants in addition to our shift charting, as well as make out charge sheets for billing purposes. There was usually limited time or thought put into individual participant's needs.

Jackie offered, "I don't know if you heard it from Margie or not, but Stacey apparently told her she thinks she's bisexual. I don't think she's brought it up with her peers yet, but maybe we could talk about the wide range of normal sexuality. You know, heterosexuality, homosexuality, and bisexuality."

The sexuality education group was one of my favorites. I had begun doing it several years previously in a former job, and when I started working at Oak Haven, I offered to a group there.

Despite all the focus in the media on sex and the sophistication our children believe they have, their knowledge of basic sexuality and the complexities of intimate relationships is seriously lacking.

Schools provide what has become known as *family life educa-tion,* yet in most cases they are seriously constrained in what they may teach. There are those who object to the discussion of birth control and those who would disallow inclusion of information about abortion. Some dislike open discussion of homosexuality, and many educators find it difficult to bring up certain topics, such as masturbation. Then there are others who object to the encouragement of abstinence on the grounds that decisions about sexual behavior are a matter of personal choice. Content aside, there is always the question of the actual qualifications of those teaching such courses.

What has always struck me is the difficulty that educators and parents alike have in having an intentional and meaningful discussion about the emotional aspects of relationships and intimacy and commitment. While it's relatively easy for many to discuss the mechanics of sex, it can be harder to discuss the intricacies of establishing and maintaining a lasting and emotionally-intimate union, the path to commitment. The stuff of *feelings*. These are the aspects of sexuality which I think that adults sometimes gloss over, believing that the young people in their lives already understand, and where family, schools, and church have been most negligent. I enjoyed exploring such things with the young people on our unit.

Unfortunately the kids didn't always enjoy exploring along with me.

All things considered, though, the group went well, and we had a lively and reasonably mature discussion of sexual norms. Stacey brought up having both male and female friends, but asked no questions and made no disclosures. When the discussion touched on bisexuality, some of the kids seemed to alternately approach and retreat from talking about the topic and there seemed to be some tension in the room, as if some were avoiding a serious discussion of a threatening topic.

Given the long-held prejudice against those with alternative sexual preferences, it's not difficult to understand the confusion young people have regarding their own and others' sexuality. I decided not to press Stacey about what Jackie had told me, and I hoped Stacey would bring it up later, when she was ready.

"Okay, guys, good work. It's time for rec ..." Before I finished speaking, chairs had been pushed back and half the kids were already out the door. "... from now 'til 8:30."

Caitlyn arrived to help Jackie supervise the kids so I could get started on the group notes. I still had to pass meds, do my regular charting, and a couple of one-to-ones. With any luck, maybe I'd clock out by 11:30 and be home in bed shortly after midnight. I was waiting for the elevator when I heard someone call my name.

"Debbi?" It was Stacey. "Do you have a minute?"

I turned and said, "Sure." I'd always make time for one of the kids.

Stacey was a pretty, spunky girl with chestnut brown hair half-way down her back. She was bright and articulate and sometimes it was easy to forget she was just fourteen. We walked slowly down the hall and then decided to sit and talk in the stairwell. It was as good a place as any, and with the other kids in the gym, we wouldn't be disturbed.

"Some of the other kids know, 'cause I already talked to them, but, um, I wanted to let you know I'm, uh, bisexual." She tossed her head and smoothed her hair with her hand, all the while keeping a steady gaze on me.

I nodded to encourage her to continue.

"I already talked to Margie about it," she continued, biting her lower lip, "and she told me maybe I'm not, but I know I am. I like guys *and* girls. And not just *like*, I mean I'm attracted to them, you know, in a romantic way." She stared at me for a moment and then seemed satisfied she had said all she wanted to say. She leaned back on her elbows as an invitation for my response.

"Do you understand why Margie said maybe you're not?" I asked. "Not because there's anything wrong with being bisexual or homosexual or even heterosexual, but because sometimes kids your age ... what are you, fourteen?" I had to be careful not to make Stacey feel I was being judgmental or was, in any way, minimizing a serious subject.

She nodded.

"... sometimes kids your age wonder about sex and have questions about their sexuality. You guys are just discovering who you are and trying to find your place in the world. You may have feelings you misunderstand or misinterpret."

She was shaking her head before I even finished. "Yeah, I know that. But I'm more mature than most kids my age. I know what my feelings are."

The Forgotten Future

"Stacey, I agree that you are very mature for your age, but because you are, you also know you have to deal with life as it is in the real world. And I'm sure you know that a lot of young people, as well as adults, have trouble dealing with homosexuality or bisexuality in any way. I think what Margie was getting at, and what I'm trying to say, is that you want to be careful not to label yourself at this early age when your feelings may very well change before you're an adult. Don't saddle yourself with a label that can cause you a lot of grief from people who don't understand or won't accept you. Continue thinking about, and exploring, your options so when you're comfortable enough with who you are …"

She smiled as if she had heard all this before. "It's okay. I just wanted staff to know that I'm bisexual and that it's no problem for me. I talked to some of the kids already, and they understand."

"Stacey, I'm really glad you came to talk to me, and it's good that you feel comfortable talking with your peers. Just remember what I said about not labeling yourself, okay? And if you need to talk some more, let us know."

"Can I go to rec, now?"

"You bet!" She turned and sprinted toward the gym, and I returned to the unit to finish up the evening's work. By the time the evening's charting and miscellaneous other paperwork were completed, the kids were in bed and lights out had long ago been called. I felt guilty because there were kids I should have spent time with but never had a chance. The next two days were my days off, and I hoped that by the time I returned, things would have slowed down a bit so the kids could get what they were there for. Help.

*   *   *   *

Report went quickly on my first day back. We finished and I returned to the nurses' office.

Robin leaned through the door and spoke quietly. "Tomorrow is Amber's sixteenth birthday, so we ordered a cake if you guys want to have it on evening shift. Her dad called today to see how she's doing, and I told him about the cake. He and her stepmom will probably come in to help her celebrate, if that's okay?"

"Yeah, sure. He doesn't come in very often. I haven't met the stepmother yet, but it would be nice if they could both be here for the cake. I know Amber says she really likes her."

The hospital usually provided cakes for patients' birthdays, but sometimes families brought in their own cakes or cupcakes to celebrate. I knew that some of the other staff didn't like them to do that, but I didn't mind. My mind had already switched over, and I was beginning to plan out the evening. Rec and visiting hours were all that were on the schedule and that meant that the kids would be bored. And restless.

Visiting hours are always a challenge.

People who work the day shift in hospitals like Oak Haven really don't understand much of what goes on during the evening shift. It's a never-ending staff debate over which shift has the most stress. Having worked both, my vote is for the evening shift. It's less structured, there are fewer support people, and the kids are tired and frustrated. Visiting hours are sometimes the straw that breaks the camel's back. This particular night was one of those camelback nights.

Only a few of the kids had visitors on any kind of a regular basis, and some of the kids never had any visitors at all. They are brought to the hospital and left. Kids are not at the top of some parents' lists.

Fifteen-year-old Emily, though, was fortunate. Both her mom and stepfather visited almost every evening and usually brought along her sixteen-year-old sister, Marianne, and her seven-year-old brother, Gary.

Emily's mom and stepfather were both teachers, and her mom was typical of many of the brighter, better-educated parents: she blamed herself for most of Emily's problems. She needed frequent reassurance from staff about her decisions on discipline and child rearing and often second-guessed herself.

When I started hourly rounds, Emily, Gary, and their stepfather were engaged in a rousing game of Yahtzee at the end of the hall. Emily's mother was once again picking Caitlyn's brain about parenting. Rounds during visiting hours are important to make sure everyone is okay, the kids aren't getting into any trouble, and the visits are under control.

The unit rule was that all the doors to patients' rooms had to remain open except at bedtime, so I was surprised to find the door to Emily's and Stacey's room closed.

"Hello?" I tapped lightly on the door. Grasping the doorknob, I pushed the door open several inches and peeked in.

I was unprepared for what I found when I opened the door. Stacey and Marianne were embracing and involved in a deep and very sensual kiss. Summoning all the professionalism I could muster, I stepped into the room and said, "Ladies, I'm sorry but you can't do that here. Stacey, you aren't even supposed to be visiting with Marianne. She's not your visitor. Marianne, you're here to visit with Emily."

I stepped back as an invitation for Marianne to leave the room, but after she passed I stepped forward to block Stacey from walking out.

"Stacey, we gotta talk. You can't do this …" I started.

"Debbi, what? What do you want me to say? I *care* for Beth. She's like me. *I don't know what to say.*" Stacey looked to be in pain, and she was pleading with me to understand.

"Stacey, it doesn't matter whether Beth is a boy or a girl. I …" but she brushed past me and was already walking down the hall toward the community room. I decided it wasn't the time to try to talk to her. Maybe later, when she was calmer and the visitors were gone.

I found Emily screaming in whispers to her mother and Caitlyn. Her stepfather was still engrossed in Yahtzee.

I figured I'd better go check things out, and as I approached them, I heard Emily hiss, "She's a whore!"

"What's going on?" I asked, looking from Emily to her mother and then back again.

"Marianne!" Emily answered, barely below a shout. "She's supposed to be visiting me, and she's in there makin' out with Stacey! She's a *whore!*" She screamed the last word, then turned on her heel, walked into her room and slammed the door.

I realized then that Marianne had come out and complained to her very unsympathetic sister. I didn't know, though, whether

Deborah Clark Ebel, R.N.

Emily was angrier about her sister's unconventional behavior or about being ignored during the visit. Probably a little of both, I decided.

Marianne stood in the corner with her arms crossed, angrily shaking her leg. Gary and Emily's stepfather hastily gathered their coats, and Emily's mother looked embarrassed about what was happening. Emily's mother said good-bye to everyone, but to no one in particular, and the family moved toward the door speaking in rapid, angry-sounding voices.

Some of the other kids and their visitors were observing and talking behind their hands about all this, while at the same time trying to appear uninterested.

"It's okay. Everything's okay," I said, as much to convince myself as to convince them. I hoped I was right.

I walked into the nurses' office and dropped into the nearest chair.

*   *   *   *

The standard unit procedure for kids returning from pass was pretty straightforward. The kids were supposed to change into pajamas in front of staff and we searched their clothing and any items that had been brought in. Then we obtained a urine specimen for pot and cocaine and had them use the Breathalyzer to check for alcohol.

Kids scheduled for their first pass were often sniggeringly teased by their peers about the "strip search" that would be done upon their return from pass, but, in fact, we didn't even watch them undress when they came back. We allowed them to change behind a bathroom stall door and pass their clothes out to us. Then we checked their clothing, shoes, and belongings, even though we knew there were still ways to sneak in whatever they might be determined to sneak in. The urine specimen and Breathalyzer, although usually done, were sometimes omitted, especially when we were busy.

On this evening, it was an assembly line as several of the kids returned from pass in rapid succession. Clothing and belongings search, urine spec, Breathalyzer.

The Forgotten Future

Kayla stood off to one side, watching. She approached and asked if she could try the Breathalyzer because she'd never had a pass and hadn't had a chance to see what it was like. I explained how it worked, but put her off and didn't let her use it.

She asked again—and again—and again—until finally, since she seemed so determined and interested, I had her draw in a deep breath and blow into the tiny tube. "Breathe, breathe, breathe … okay."

I looked at the digital readout and was shocked to find she had a positive reading for alcohol. A very positive reading. *Shit.*

Our eyes met, and she exploded into laughter. "What …?" I asked, gullibly.

"Hairspray," she beamed, and pulled a pump bottle from behind her back. "I sprayed it in my mouth." She opened wide and pointed, as if there were something there to see. "I just wondered what would happen." She took a quick dancing step backward to bask in the success of her deception.

Kayla didn't use drugs or alcohol, but a lot of the kids who were into substances used seemingly innocuous over-the-counter drugs such as Coricidin Cough and Cold (known as triple C), Robitussin, or NyQuil to get high. Parents rarely suspected their children of abusing these medications and did not realize that some teens and preteens were drinking upwards of two or three bottles a day of such liquids. Staff at Oak Haven and similar hospitals knew about the dangers of over-the-counter meds and didn't allow these or similar products to be brought onto the unit. Even mouthwashes containing alcohol were prohibited. Hairspray was another story entirely, however.

Kayla had used the hairspray to see if we could catch the alcohol on her breath and what we would do if we did. Her actions earned her room restriction and a writing assignment about what was inappropriate about her actions. Then we confiscated all the hairspray on the unit and decided that we would have to look into revising the hospital policy once again regarding what was, and was not, allowed on the unit.

*　　*　　*　　*

Deborah Clark Ebel, R.N.

One of the more challenging things about working with adolescents is how quickly their moods can change. Emotions run hot and cold among teenagers, and even on their best days, what you see is not what you'll get five minutes later. You never know what to expect.

Lights-out was fast approaching, and Caitlyn directed everyone to their respective rooms. I was preparing bedtime meds when I heard screams from the hall.

I ran into the hall and found Caitlyn trying to break up a fight between Emily and Stacey. The girls were shouting and calling each other names and clawing and hitting at each other. Stacey, the more athletic of the two, seemed to be the aggressor, while Emily seemed to be the more imaginative at name-calling. Emily's lower lip was bleeding following a blow from Stacey's right fist, and her fingers were coiled through Stacey's hair, tugging hard. A couple of the other kids were trying to help Caitlyn pull the two apart; the rest seemed to be enjoying the action. Robert and Meghan and Amber were huddled in the corner staring.

I rushed in and blocked Stacey while Caitlyn pushed Emily out of Stacey's reach. I couldn't get a good hold on Stacey alone, so Caitlyn assisted with the takedown and helped me lower her to the ground as gently as we could. "Watch her head! Watch out … her leg … don't let her kick you!"

The two girls continued screeching at each other. Emily stood to the side, taunting Stacey, while Stacey, now on the floor, angrily answered Emily's jeers.

"Bitch!"

"Whore!"

"Cunt!"

"I hate you!"

"I hate you more!"

"I'm going to *kill* you!"

"Bitch!"

Caitlyn and I both yelled for Emily to go into her room—*Now!*—and for the other kids to go into their rooms. Some did and some didn't. Typical.

The Forgotten Future

Although we had Stacey under control on the floor, our dilemma now was what to do with her. Every time we eased up on our hold, she started struggling again, even if she had promised she wouldn't.

Stacey shifted slightly, and Caitlyn made an "O-o-o-o" sound. Stacey lifted her head mere inches and said, very genuinely, "Oh, I'm sorry, Caitlyn. Did I hurt you?" Stacey wasn't totally out of control, as was obvious by her concern over possibly hurting Caitlyn. She was using our restraint, as many kids do in similar circumstances, to impose control on herself so she didn't have to use her own inner mechanisms. Still, every time we loosened our hold, she would start struggling again.

At the other end of the hall, Emily's rage seemed to have cooled. I could see her whispering conspiratorially with Dea and Amber.

Caitlyn and I were the only staff on the unit, and since we were both restraining Stacy, there was no one available to call for backup to monitor and supervise the rest of the kids. In the past, a few of us had voiced concern that something like this might happen, and now we were in the middle of it.

The phone in the nurses' office rang six or seven times and then fell silent. We stayed on the floor, holding Stacey, for half an hour or more. One by one, the rest of the kids, including Emily, seemed to tire of the show and went to their rooms and, we hoped, to bed.

Stacey was slowly regaining control, and we asked for promises that she would stay away from Emily and not fight or attack us or Emily if we released her. We told her that she would have to sleep in the seclusion room, and she agreed to our conditions. Then, as we stood and headed toward the seclusion area, we held tight onto Stacey's arms for everyone's safety.

As we walked past the room she shared with Emily, though, we heard Emily shout out, "I'm going to kill you, Bitch! You just wait. I'm going to fuckin' kill you!" Stacey strained against our hold and yelled back at Emily, "C'mon, 'ho! Bring it on!" We tightened our grasp and kept walking.

It was 12:45 in the early morning hours before we finally

walked out into the clear, crisp night. It had taken hours to quell the agitation on the unit, get the necessary doctor's orders for Stacy's seclusion, and complete the charting and incident reports. It had been an exhausting shift, physically and emotionally.

I kept thinking about Stacey. I couldn't get the vision of her pleading eyes out of my mind. Caitlyn and I talked for a few minutes in the parking lot, and then I bade her good night and started the short drive home.

After I pulled into my driveway and turned off the car engine, I allowed the quiet darkness to surround me. I ruminated on the value of our work at Oak Haven, wondering what good we were doing, what we were accomplishing. However clichéd it might sound, I became a nurse to help people and to ease their suffering. I knew that I was a good nurse and had made a positive difference in the lives of many people. I wanted to believe that I was *still* making a difference, but sometimes the administration's health-care-is-a-business-and-we-have-to-save-dollars-wherever-we-can-and-let's-start-by-making-cuts-in-staffing choices and decisions were so oppressive that any good the staff was able to do was distorted by what we were *not* able to achieve.

I had for months been quietly questioning whether psychiatric hospitals like Oak Haven were accomplishing anything near what the public believes and expects. Were the kids in our care truly benefitting from their confinements or were they more often than not being routinely prescribed psychotropic medications and being unnecessarily exposed to those more seriously behaviorally and emotionally-disordered than themselves?

Tiredness suddenly overwhelmed me, and I couldn't, didn't want to, think anymore. I knew I wasn't going to solve the world's problems this night, so I decided that I might as well get some sleep. I walked up the steps to my door, glad to be home.

*   *   *   *

As soon as all admission assessments and pertinent outside histories on a patient are received, the treatment team begins planning for discharge. Depending on the needs of the patient and the family, one of several things happens at discharge:

A patient may return home, either with or without follow-up mental health treatment.

A patient may be placed in a therapeutic foster home or group home.

A patient may be transferred to a long-term residential treatment
center.

Meghan's mother was willing to have her return home to live, but despite the family's problems, Child Protective Services did not feel there was any reason to become involved.

The problem was that Meghan refused to go home. She saw living with her mother as an untenable proposition and one from which she would very likely flee within a short time. Her grandmother's home was no longer an option for a number of reasons, and she realized that returning to her former living situation with Evan and Dirk was neither healthy nor safe. She didn't have any suggestions, but at the same time she was unwilling to accept the options available to her. So, for the time being, she would remain at Oak Haven.

She didn't like that idea either.

*   *   *   *

"Debbi, it really reeks down there now. It's like sick or something, and we're trying to have my birthday cake." Amber was the third person to complain this shift of a foul odor at the end of the hall. Maintenance had been called to check and quickly ruled out the more obvious possible causes. There was no backed-up plumbing, no unusual odors from the ventilation system, trash cans were emptied, and they had been unable to track down the source of the stink.

"They're still checking things out, Amber. I know it smells bad, but just keep the windows open. That's the best I can offer." *They* weren't really checking anything, because *they* didn't have a clue what the heck it was. I think they were just hoping the smell would go away.

As the evening passed, I forgot all about the smell, or maybe I just got used to it. In any event, it was far from my mind when I heard a loud, *"Holy Mother of Jesus! These kids ... these kids!"* from room 407.

Lydia, one of the housekeepers, had gone to clean the room after its occupant was discharged, and she now emerged, face red, hands out to her sides. The front of her blue utility uniform was wet with a large, dark yellow-brown area. She spoke rapidly in a foreign language.

I didn't understand the words, but I got the idea. To say she went ballistic doesn't come close to describing her rage. As I quickly moved toward her, she recovered enough English to tell me to look in the nightstand drawer in 407. She smelled bad. So did the room.

The drawer stood wide open, liquid standing rancid inside the drawer. Lydia stood behind me, pointing. "Look at that!" she ranted. "It is *disgusting*! I will not clean this up."

I had to agree. It *was* disgusting. The drawer, approximately ten inches wide, twelve inches long, and six inches deep, was filled to the brim with sour, stinking, putrid urine and feces.

Jared, a quiet, bespectacled fifteen-year-old who had been discharged earlier in the day, had evidently been using the drawer as his personal toilet for a week or more, possibly longer. Had he not been discharged, Lydia wouldn't have been cleaning his room. If she hadn't been cleaning his room, we might not have found the drawer until who knows when.

But we did find it, and it was a first. Housekeeping had a mess to clean up, and they weren't happy. For the next week, though, the boys enjoyed a few laughs with, "I gotta *pee!*" and pulling out their nightstand drawers.

*   *   *   *

The unit was busy, and time passed quickly. The unit census was high; the acuity was higher. Several admissions and discharges took place, and the unit continued on its course. Kayla was troubled over her impending out-of-state move, Meghan was becoming more aggressive, and Stacey and Emily continued to verbally abuse and threaten each other. Robert had begun flirting with both Dea and Teresa, and it looked like Teresa might be interested. Our big question mark, however, remained Stacey.

We were all concerned about Stacey. She seemed to become angrier and more threatening every day, yet she wasn't willing to talk to anyone about what was going on. Emily would be discharged in a few days, and we hoped that would defuse Stacey so she could start working on whatever was causing her depression. The other side of the coin was that if Stacey wasn't able to keep her anger under control and assure us she wouldn't take out her aggression on Emily or anyone else, we would have to think about moving her into our close observation unit (COU). As it was, we allowed her to attend select groups with close monitoring and with her promise to keep herself under control.

Thursday evening passed uneventfully, and after drug ed we directed the kids to the group room for the evening's Wrap Up.

Teresa and Meghan came to the nurses' office. Teresa looked upset and attempted to convince Jackie that she needed to use the phone for a quick last-minute phone call to her mom.

Robert and Dea stood in the hall, engaged in what looked like a serious conversation, and I wondered if that was why Teresa was upset. I hoped there wasn't any pairing-off going on, even though I knew better than to seriously think that. Hormones in hospitals where adolescent males and females are housed together seem to ooze out of the walls. This was especially true when there was a Lothario like Robert on the scene.

The kids straggled into the group room, and we were several minutes late getting started. Teresa volunteered to run the meeting and started by reciting the Serenity Prayer. I noticed that Amber was missing, and I slipped out to ask her to join us.

Her room was dark as I entered. Despite the fact that it was close to 9:30, no lights were on, not even the faint glow from the supposed-to-be-on nightlight. Nothing unusual there; it was either burned out or it had been removed by one of the kids and hadn't been replaced.

I heard muffled crying from the corner.

Deborah Clark Ebel, R.N.

"Amber, are you there? It's Debbi. What's wrong?" I continued cautiously into the room and found Amber curled up in the corner on top of the nightstand. Knees drawn up, head down, hair damp from sweat and tears. She didn't answer. I stood beside her, and began to gently rub her upper back.

"Amber, hon, what's the matter? What's going on?"

Her shoulders heaved as she tried hard to keep the sobs in. I continued to rub her shoulders and remained silent for several minutes. Finally, I said, "Amber, I need to know why you're crying. You have to talk to me."

Her face was wet and puffy when she finally looked up. "It's Robert," she said between sniffles. "He made me do things …"

My first thought was, "Oh, shit!" Instinct told me it had to be sexual. Those damn hormones. My second thought was concern for Amber. She was obviously upset, and if Robert was sneaking into her room and doing things to her … My third thought was *incident report.*

I quickly ran the past several days over in my mind and wondered what cues I might have missed. I hadn't even realized they were an item. I thought he was making his moves on Teresa, or maybe Dea. If he and Amber had gotten together, especially *this* close together, I sure hoped it hadn't happened during one of my shifts. I had to find out *what* had happened and *when* and *where*. I needed information. I could ask questions, but I needed to let *her* tell *me*. I couldn't lead her on.

"Okay, Amber. I know you're upset, but we need to talk. Robert made you do things? Can you tell me what things?"

She began, hesitatingly at first, until finally the whole story came out. Mostly, she talked and I listened, although I occasionally asked questions to clarify things that weren't clear to me. We stayed there in the corner of her darkened room for a long time.

She told me that she liked Robert a lot and was thrilled when he invited her into his room. She hoped he would ask her to "go out" with him. At first they had just kissed and touched, but by the third day things had gone further. Much further. She said he forced her to come to his room every morning during the change-of-shift report. For fifteen minutes, no one was assigned to watch the hall and they had complete privacy, except for Robert's roommate, Jerry. All she had to do was run straight across the hall to Robert's room.

"His room? In Robert's room?" I had to make sure I had this right. I felt like I was missing something—I just didn't understand how he was making her come into his room. Threats? Manipulation? What was he doing? Amber offered no specifics on *how*, but she was adamant that he was forcing her to do this in his room.

Being able to talk about what had happened, even for just a few minutes, had allowed Amber to settle down a bit. I got a cool, damp washcloth from her bathroom and wiped her face. At very stressful times, the adolescents became just like little children and needed some mothering. We hugged, and I told her I was going to talk to Robert. Tonight. That she didn't have to go to his room again.

Jackie looked up as I walked into the nurses' office. Wrap Up was over. "You were in there a long time. What's goin' on?"

I sighed, "It's Amber and Robert. We have problems. *Big* problems." I filled her in on what Amber had told me, and we discussed how best to confront Robert. All the kids were in bed, so Caitlyn could handle the unit while Jackie and I were in with Robert. We decided to talk to him in the conference room.

*   *   *   *

Robert shuffled into the conference room and slumped into the swivel chair by the window. "What? What'd I do?" he asked, sounding as if he didn't really care what our answer was. Most of our kids automatically assumed they were in trouble any time an adult wanted to talk to them. In this case, he was right. He *was* in trouble.

He had a smile that could melt hearts. Tall and strikingly handsome, at thirteen he already displayed the polished poise and air of self-assurance that in a few short years would have women vying for his attention.

And he was a con man.

His official diagnosis was conduct disorder, but he demonstrated serious antisocial personality traits. People with antisocial

Deborah Clark Ebel, R.N.

personality disorder exhibit behavior that chronically manipulates, exploits, or violates the rights of others. This behavior is often criminal, but a diagnosis of antisocial personality disorder cannot technically be made until the patient is at least eighteen years old. Robert was young, but he was well on his way. He met all the criteria except for age.

We had seen many youngsters with an unofficial diagnosis of antisocial charm their way through treatment, but Robert was good. He was *very* good. Look out world, lock up your daughters and hide the keys to your cars.

"Robert, we need to talk. I spent some time with Amber earlier tonight, and she told me some things that really concern me. Some things about you." I looked straight into his eyes.

He knew I was serious.

"Yeah, well, so what? What'd she say?" His attitude was that this was an inconvenience, not that there was any real problem. He twisted and turned the chair from side to side. It squeaked.

I chose my words carefully. "What I want to know, Robert, what I need to know, is your side of the story. Amber told me some things about what the two of you have been doing sexually, and I'm concerned."

We bantered back and forth for about ten minutes, with my being circumspect and Robert sounding me out to find out how much I really knew. He was smart and wasn't about to be bluffed into saying something we didn't already know. He continued slouching, but a grin slowly spread across his face.

"Whatever she said," he said quietly.

"Excuse me?" Jackie asked. We worked well together. She picked up where I left off. Not quite good-cop, bad-cop, but it was close.

"Whatever she said we did, we did." He glanced away as he spoke. Eye contact was a little harder for him now. He turned the swivel chair around in a circle to avoid looking straight at me.

"Robert, how do you know what she said? We need you to tell us what happened. We need to hear you say it in your own words." Watching him reminded me how very young he was.

"I can't." He blushed, and turned away.

"Robert, you have to tell us." Jackie leaned forward in her chair.

I wondered if he had any idea what Amber had told me. If he did, I couldn't imagine he would be so willing to give her control of the situation by admitting to "whatever she said".

"I can't say it. I can't say the words. Whatever she said, it's true. I did it." He squirmed in his chair and started to look the thirteen-year-old he was.

He continued swiveling the chair. I reached out and put my hand on the arm of the chair and stopped it. We had been at this for a long time and still weren't getting anywhere. "Robert, if you're old enough to do it, you're old enough to say the words."

"C'mon. I can't. I just can't say the words. I can do it, I just can't talk about it."

"Look, Robert, I know what Amber has said, and we have a very definite problem here. I need to hear your side of the story. From you." I was trying hard to keep the exasperation out of my voice, but we were just going around and around in circles. "Can you use other words to tell me?"

He thought a minute and then answered, "I can tell you *sort* of what we did." He went back to twisting the chair from side to side.

"Okay. Tell us *sort of.*" Jackie sounded edgy. It was getting late, and we needed to move on or call it quits for the night.

"Well, she did to me, you know, what you would do to an ice cream cone. I was the ice cream cone." He looked down.

"An ice cream cone?" The imagery was certainly unique …

"Yeah, well, she came into my room and licked and sucked me, uh, my privates. She wanted to." He was blushing, but was finally looking at us and seemed a little more comfortable now that he was talking. Then he looked away and twisted in his chair again.

"Amber said you made her do it."

"What?" he yelled as he twirled around and sat straight up in his chair. "I *didn't!* She came into my room; she asked me to do it. You can ask Jerry! She wanted him to do it, too!"

"So you're telling me she approached you first and asked to have oral sex with you?" I felt like the Grand Inquisitor. Nursing school hadn't prepared me for this.

Deborah Clark Ebel, R.N.

"Yes! You can ask Jerry! He'll tell you. And then we had regular sex! Her and me! It was all her idea."

We talked for awhile longer, and then I told Robert that the day staff would discuss things with him further in the morning. Obviously, there would be consequences for what was very inappropriate interaction between two young teens, but even beyond that, I knew the fact that this had happened while they were both in the care and custody of the hospital was going to be a major problem in the eyes of their parents. In the meantime, we told Robert that he was to have no contact at all with Amber.

* * * *

I hurriedly slipped into a chair in the conference room the next afternoon to take report from the day shift. "Sorry guys." I grabbed a report sheet and picked through the desk drawer trying to find a black pen that worked. "It was just so beautiful outside today that I lost track of time. I envy you … you get to enjoy the afternoon sun … unless you want to stay and I'll leave?"

"Not a chance," groaned Robin. "It's been a real mess here all day. You were here last night, so you know what I'm talking about."

Yeah, I knew all right. I could only imagine what had gone on regarding Amber and Robert, from the administrative level on down. I was sure it had gone from the unit staff to the doctor to the director of nursing, up to the administration, back down to the director of nursing, back to the unit staff, and without a doubt the kids all knew about it by now. "Okay," I said, "we might as well get started."

"All right, in room 401A we have Amy J. She's fifteen, Dr. Evans' patient, and her diagnosis is oppositional defiant disorder. She slept all night, but today has been a difficult one. She had a family therapy session, and her mother told her she can't come back home to live. Amy took it pretty hard, but she's probably going to be much better off going to live in a group home. Tomorrow Margie is going to meet with her and explore her options."

There was little else Robin could tell me about Amy. She was a good kid and I hoped things would work out for her. Her mother had a way of bringing out the worst in her, and having met her mother on several occasions, I could understand it completely. She brought out the worst in me, too.

"Room 401B is empty; room 402A is Meghan R., Dr. Carmichael's patient, in with polysubstance abuse and conduct disorder. Her behavior is getting worse. She doesn't want to be here and is demanding that we let her leave. Watch her for possible AWOL. 402B is empty. 403A was Emily. She was discharged back home to her parents. Thank God. 403B is Stacey D., Dr. Evans' patient in with major depression. She's out on pass with her dad 'til about 5:30."

Report continued uneventfully until we got to room 408 and Amber. Robin leaned back in her chair and drew in a deep breath. "Let me tell you about Amber," she said, shaking her head.

"She woke up early this morning all cheerful, like nothing had happened. Connie went in to talk to her, and then Dr. Evans showed up. The three of them talked for about an hour and a half, and guess what? She admitted that the blowjobs were *her* idea! And the sex. Apparently she does things like this to get guys to "like" her and "go out" with her." Robin shook her head in disbelief. "When I was thirteen, I was still playing with dolls!"

"So Robert just sort of took advantage of the situation? Sort of like, don't look a gift horse in the mouth?" ventured Caitlyn. Our eyes met and we broke up over the unintended pun.

We knew there was nothing funny about the situation, nothing funny at all. But working within such an outrageous environment often brought out humor from the far side.

"Right," said Robin, "but even though she was the initiator, the administration thought it would be best to get Robert out of here ASAP, just in case he thought he could get the same treatment from someone else. They transferred him out to Longmeadow about an hour ago. Amber has apparently been sexually active since she was eleven and really craves male attention. Her dad is really bent out of shape about Robert, though, and is thinking about bringing charges for rape even though Robert's only thirteen, himself. He's also talking about suing the hospital."

Deborah Clark Ebel, R.N.

Robert and Amber were both still just kids and didn't really understand the possible consequences of their behavior. I didn't blame Amber's dad for being angry, but maybe he also needed to look at what's really going on with his daughter. Why does she feel she has to do sexual favors to get guys to pay attention to her? She certainly had some serious problems; that's why she was in the hospital. But we weren't a locked unit in the strictest sense of the word, nor was it single-sex, and the kids weren't watched constantly. It's easy for parents to lay blame on others, even though they haven't been able to control their kids at home. Nevertheless, if I were the parent of one of these kids, I would expect my child to be in a much more strictly-controlled environment than we provided. I guess I would expect a lot more of just about every aspect of the hospitalization.

We finished report, and the evening began. I stood to start rounds, wondering silently how close parents' expectations of psychiatric hospitalization is to reality. I knew that the parents really didn't have a clue.

Chapter 4
Lost Innocence

I had just finished speaking on the phone when I heard a commotion, a shriek from somewhere down the hall. Caitlyn cried out, "Can I get some help down here? Call Dr. Strong!"

Pausing for the five seconds or so that it took to do an overhead page of "Dr. Strong to the adolescent unit! Dr. Strong to the adolescent unit!" I ran to the utility room and grabbed the safety coat.

When I arrived at room 403, I found Stacey standing on her bed, screaming hysterically and ripping the curtains from the windows. The desk chair was overturned; paper and trash were strewn about the room. The trashcan was lying on its side underneath a new hole in the wall.

I stopped and stood just outside the doorway.

"I don't know what's going on," Caitlyn said, breathlessly. "She came back from pass, and everything seemed to be okay. Her dad said the pass went well, and they went to McDonald's to eat. She seemed happy. And then I heard this!"

Stacey was doubled over, fists clinched. She wailed, over and over, "I want to die!"

Apparently things hadn't gone so well after all.

We needed emergency staff, and response to our Dr. Strong was good. Looking around, I saw there were five or six people standing at the ready in the hall, including two males.

Deborah Clark Ebel, R.N.

Speaking softly, I kept my hands in full view at my sides so as not to be a threat. "Stacey? *Stacey.* What's going on? Can you come down so we can talk?"

I didn't want Stacey up on the bed because I didn't want her to fall and get hurt and I also didn't want her in a position where a purposeful or a random kick could connect and injure someone if we had to take her down. And I didn't think taking her down was a matter of if, but when.

"Debbi, *honest to God,* don't come in here! I don't want to hurt you, and I swear to God I'll hurt you if you come in. Don't come any closer!" Her voice was hoarse from screaming, and tears streamed down her face. She looked scared, like a caged animal.

I knew she really didn't want to hurt me. She didn't want to hurt anyone. But when patients are angry or scared, they sometimes do things that they would never do otherwise, and while I thought I would be safe, I couldn't take a chance. "It's okay, Stacey, it's okay. I'm not coming any closer. We just need to know that you're okay. Can we sit down and talk? I'm really worried about you up there on the bed. I'm afraid you'll fall or something. Come on down and we'll talk. Nobody is going to hurt you."

I really cared about Stacey. Working with patients in a setting as intense as a psychiatric hospital, one comes to know patients more intimately than do their families, their loved ones, even than they know themselves. And invariably, just as in life on the outside, there are some patients you connect with more than others. Stacey and I had that kind of connection, and sometimes I had to struggle to maintain the professional boundary my job demanded.

"No, Debbi, I can't! You don't understand! I just want to die! Please let me die!" She was screaming and losing any remaining control fast. It was time to make a decision.

There are times that patients, given a little extra time and support to work through their immediate crisis, are able to calm themselves enough so that no extreme measures are necessary. I knew that we were far beyond such a time with Stacey. There were a couple of beds available in the COU, and in my judgment Stacey needed to be there, even if only for a short period of time. We could not maintain a safe environment in the open unit with her in this condition, and I was sure Dr. Carmichael would order the transfer when told of her condition. The hospital nursing supervisor arrived, and after assessing the situation, she left to call Dr. Carmichael to get orders.

It was time to move, and I turned toward the MHTs and gave them a barely perceptible nod. They carried the green canvas safety coat into the room and started spreading it out on the floor.

A safety coat, sometimes called a body bag, is commonly used to restrain adolescents and adults who are deemed to be at risk of harming themselves or others. Much more than what people think of as a straight jacket, it covers the out-of-control patient from over the shoulders to over the toes. It is made of a heavy material similar to that used in old military duffel bags.

The out-of-control patient is placed on the opened safety coat, usually fighting and yelling, and their shoes, eyeglasses and any necklaces, bracelets and watches are removed. The clothing pockets are checked to remove any items such as pencils, earrings, etc. that might be used by the patient to harm himself while restrained or which might "poke" into his body by pressure from the coat.

The patient's arms are then straightened as much as possible. Wooden slats buried within the canvas are checked, and the coat is wrapped around the patient's body from both sides, covering the patient from the neck down to and over the feet. The body-length, heavy-duty zipper is then secured, and heavy buckles are applied to completely restrain the patient.

The patient is usually then placed on a stretcher or hospital bed and wheeled to a seclusion room or other safe area.

Because use of the safety coat is a high-risk measure, once restrained, the patient must never be left alone, not even for a short time. Monitoring of the patient's temperature, blood pressure, level of alertness, circulation, position, and general status is done and recorded on forms that become part of the patient's permanent chart. The patient must be offered food and water at least every two hours. This monitoring is generally done by MHTs, with the nurse checking on the patient hourly, or more often if there appears to be a problem.

Only a licensed staff member, i.e., a doctor or a registered nurse, can call for the mechanical restraint of a patient. A MHT cannot make that decision. If a decision is made to apply restraints and a doctor is not present, a registered nurse must call the physician as soon as possible to obtain an order for the restraints. A physician is required to physically examine the restrained patient within one hour of the initiation of the restraint and at that time, orders for the restraint itself, as well as orders indicating the length of time the restraint may be continued, must be written.

Being placed in restraints can be a frightening experience for someone who is already out of control, so it's important that only one person speak calmly to the patient and provide reassurances while restraints are being applied. Despite what some patients believe, an order for restraints is given only after all other measures to help the patient regain control have been exhausted. It is precisely because patients are not thinking clearly and do not fully appreciate that they are jeopardizing the safety of everyone—themselves, peers, and staff—that such measures are necessary. While the best possible scenario would be to continue working to help a patient calm down for whatever length of time it might take to avoid extreme measures, in reality that cannot be done with limited staff and a full unit to be managed.

I stepped forward and spoke softly, "Stacey, I need you to come down off the bed now. You can't continue like this; it isn't safe for you or for us. I would prefer that you get down now and walk down the hall with me under your own power, but if you can't do that, we can help you."

"No! Don't come any closer! I swear to god ..." and she let out another spine-chilling scream.

I nodded to my team and said simply, "Okay." They moved in and grabbed her two legs and two arms, lifting her off the bed and placing her, kicking and screaming, cursing and damning, onto the safety coat and began to zip and strap her in. I wished she would just stop—that she would regain control—but that didn't happen. I hated what we were doing, but I knew we had to do it for everyone's safety.

She screamed, "Stop it, you mother fuckers! Don't hold me down ... let me go ..." again ending with a soul-destroying shriek.

The Forgotten Future

Despite her gymnast-like moves, she was quickly restrained and lifted onto a stretcher to be wheeled to the COU. I ran ahead to clear the way and unlock the doors. The rest of the team followed, wheeling a terrified and screaming Stacey through the hall.

I knew that this was probably having a devastating effect on some of the kids, and we would have to give them a brief explanation at some point. If I felt this bad about the situation, I knew some of them probably felt worse.

Once inside the COU, Stacey was no longer my patient. My responsibility for her was relinquished to Diana, the COU nurse. My care for her, however, was not. I stood in the doorway wondering what had happened—not just tonight, but in the past—to cause this. What had someone done to this child to bring her to this state, and what kind of society tolerated conditions that would allow any child to be destroyed this way? She wasn't crazy, neither in a psychiatric sense nor from a layman's perspective. She was, however, in a great deal of trouble and a great deal of pain.

I wanted to take a break, to take a few minutes to gather my thoughts, but there just wasn't time. I returned to the nurses' office and thought about the phone calls I had to make, the orders to be taken off, Stacey's belongings to gather and transfer, and the eleven other teenagers to comfort and reassure. What had just transpired had to be processed with the rest of the staff and documented on several different levels. With only two mental health techs to assist with the kids, most of it was my responsibility and I could only do what I could do. My thoughts were that once again the kids were being short-changed.

Caitlyn and Jackie were good with the kids, but they were limited in what they could do. Despite their good intentions, it was impossible for them to connect with all the kids and, anyway, their role wasn't that of therapist. Ideally, professional staff should have been available to work with the kids and talk about what they had just witnessed. The reality of the situation was that I was tied up on the phone and drowning in paperwork.

Just before I gave the end-of-shift report, I was able to steal away from the desk briefly and stopped in to see a few kids whom I thought might be having a particularly difficult time. They wanted to know what had happened and why. And what would happen to Stacey now. Tempering reassurance with respect for Stacey's privacy and a great deal of honest uncertainty, I answered their questions the best that I could, all the while wishing I had someone to answer my own questions.

When I left the unit that evening, I paused at the large safety-glass window of the COU and peered in. Stacey's door was closed, but I wondered how she was, if she was asleep. My eyes burned, and I felt a lone tear escape and roll down my cheek. I reached up and touched the glass and wished her a peaceful night, hoping that I, too, might have the same, and slowly walked toward the exit door.

*   *   *   *

The phone must have rung for a long time, woven as it was into my dream. When I finally emerged from my slumber and realized that I had to answer it, I fumbled at the nightstand and answered, "Hello?"

"Deb? This is Connie at work. I hope I didn't wake you, but I just wanted to let you know how Stacey is doing." She sounded tired. "I knew you would be worried about her."

"Oh, hi Connie. That's okay. I should've been up anyway. How is she?"

"Well, she had a rough night. They gave her Ativan and Thorazine IM a couple of times, but that didn't even touch her. She's still really agitated." Connie paused and sighed before continuing. "Then this morning she disclosed to Margie that her dad has been raping her since she was eight. She says that when he took her out on pass yesterday, he threatened to hurt her if she told. Apparently he thought we were getting too close to learning what has been going on."

"Oh, *no!*" I remembered how distressed Stacey had become over the past weeks and how distraught she was last night.

"Yeah, well, that's what she says, anyway. Margie is filing a report with Child Protective Services today, so they'll do an investigation. And Dr. Carmichael wants her to stay in the COU for a few days."

"Oh, god yes. If you had seen her last night … There's just no way she can be on the open unit."

"No, you're right. She can't. Hold on …" I heard muffled conversation, then, "Hey, listen, are you working tonight?"

"Yeah, I am."

"Okay, I have to get over and talk to Margie again, but maybe I'll see you when you come in. I just wanted to let you know about what has happened before you came in."

I hung up and leaned back on my pillows. I was glad Connie had called, but I was really disturbed to learn about Stacey's abuse and that her dad was her abuser. It must have been a tremendous conflict for her to have to protect her dad when he was the one who was hurting her.

Part of my frustration that morning, even my anger, was that none of us had suspected that her father was molesting her. None of the usual signs or cues seemed to be there, nothing in the behavior of either had pointed to an abusive relationship.

I rolled over and sat on the side of the bed with my head in my hands. Sexual abuse can be a devastating experience, and when it is complicated by incest it's even more so. So many kids these days have to cope with such abuse, yet they do a heroic job confronting and recovering from what has happened. As with many horrors survived, however, some grow up using their abuse as an excuse for everything that ever goes wrong in their lives.

It can never be erased. It happened. It was wrong. But while the terrible events cannot be changed, in order to move on to a happy and successful life, the survivor at some point has to decide to move on and not let the perpetrator take any more of their life— not to forget what has happened, but to learn how to live and thrive and grow and have a fulfilling life.

Stacey, though—would she be able to move on? She was bright and had an inner strength that had carried her this far. I wanted to believe she could, and would, work this through and come out stronger on the other side. But I just didn't know. Who ever knows?

I sat and thought about all the kids I had worked with over the years. After a long time, I stood and walked into the kitchen. I had a headache.

*   *   *   *

One of the more challenging cases for me emotionally occurred shortly after I moved into the field of psychiatric nursing. Billy was a small and rather fragile-looking thirteen-year old, mischievous as Puck, with a face ready to burst into a giant smile at the slightest provocation. His parents brought him to the psychiatric unit where I worked with complaints about being unable to "do anything" with him.

The younger of two children, Billy initially appeared to have a very close relationship with his parents. His father, a burly and hard-working truck driver, and his mother, a dark and strikingly beautiful homemaker, acknowledged that they had "old-fashioned" expectations of their children and were concerned because recently Billy had been skipping school and running away. They wanted help for their only son before things got out of hand. It sounded good.

Until Billy began losing control and had to be physically restrained on a daily basis.

Until Billy escalated and required restraint in a safety coat two or three or sometimes even four times a day.

Until that same little boy sobbed and pleaded with Connie as she sat by his side, "Mommy, don't let him hit me anymore, please, Mommy!" and we broke into tears because *in his mind he was there in that basement* and there was nothing we could do except be there and watch him suffer.

Dissociative episodes are adaptive responses to traumatic situations such as childhood physical, sexual, or physical abuse during which a person feels psychologically threatened. When experiencing a dissociative episode, the person "switches off" psychologically—dissociates—from the traumatic experience as a way to deal with thoughts, emotions, sensations, or memories that are too overwhelming to handle. In other words, as a way of coping with whatever the patient is experiencing in real time or in his mind, he is able to pull his conscious self away from the situation at hand.

Child Protective Services investigated our concerns about possible abuse, and Billy's dad admitted he might have used a bat to scare young Bill once, but he had never actually hit him and would *never, ever, do such a thing again, no sir, no ma'am, never in a million years*. Child Protective Services closed the file, but no one at the hospital believed Billy's father for a minute, for we had seen Billy's terror. A short time later Billy returned home and we never heard from him again.

My experience with Billy was the beginning of the end of any remaining innocence I had about children and families. Seeing his torment within the context of our—*my*—deeply-felt inability to help him in any way gave way to a profound sense of powerlessness. I cried about it off and on for days, usually in the shower, always in a place where my own children couldn't see. Sometimes they knew I was upset and asked what was wrong. I could only mumble, "I can't talk about it" and busy myself with some household task so they wouldn't see the tears welling in my eyes. Even today, years later, I have trouble thinking about it, speaking about it, writing about it.

If Billy was the beginning of the end of my innocence, Stacey carried me further down the path.

She remained in the close observation unit and deteriorated further, screaming and thrashing, kicking and scratching, biting and clawing herself because she was "bad". The police questioned her about her allegations, and her father was arrested and charged. Stacey felt responsible and declared to everyone that it was all her fault.

She loved her father; she hated her father. She wanted to kill him; she despised herself for destroying him.

She was medicated. Repeatedly. Nothing worked. The most a 2 mg injection of Ativan or even 100 mg of Thorazine would do was cause her to slow down and doze off for a couple of hours. So many meds were tried, so little relief. She was in four-point restraints for the greater part of weeks.

Sometimes the restraints were removed, and she was able to sit in the COU community room with one-to-one supervision and draw pictures, play cards, watch television, or eat her meals. Then, suddenly, she would be overcome with self-loathing and anger and become menacing, violent, out-of-control. Once, during a standoff, she stood screaming and yelling and held a chair in the air threatening to hit the first person who came close. She glanced away for a split-second, and one of the nurses lunged forward and took the chair away before anyone was hurt.

We held her down, sometimes as many as six or eight of us, and put her into four-point restraints. She kicked and screamed as we pulled and pressed until she was strapped, splayed to the bed. Invariably, some member of the staff would try to calm her by saying, "It's okay, Stacey, just be still. We're not going to hurt you. It's okay", and then we realized how much that reminded her of her father telling her to "just lie still, it's okay, I'm not going to hurt you …"

A major concern when keeping a patient in four-point restraints for any length of time is the maintenance of proper circulation to the hands and to the feet. Each restraint must be removed on a rotating basis. Beginning with one of the ankles, the cuff is removed, the ankle massaged and circulation checked and the restraint reapplied. A half-hour later, the opposite side's wrist is done, then the same side ankle and then the opposite wrist. In this way we can ensure circulation is adequate and there are no sores or other irritations caused by the cuffs.

Sometimes, on Stacey's good days, I would sit with her in the community room and she would ask if she was bad. She questioned whether somehow she was responsible for having been molested. She believed that if she had not told about her abuse that everything would be okay and she would be back in the center of a loving, caring family. Her paternal grandparents agreed with her. We didn't let them visit again.

Her father was released from jail on bail, but wasn't allowed to visit. Valentine's Day came, and he sent her a beautiful, romantic, and totally inappropriate card. She went back into restraints..

Sometimes, on her worst days, I was assigned to the COU to do a one-to-one with Stacey. The dim overhead light cast eerie shadows on the walls, the floors, the bed, her life. I listened as she moaned and wrenched and pulled. On more than one occasion, she managed to slip a tiny wrist out of one of the restraints and quicker-than-lightening tried to unbuckle the other wrist before I noticed. She begged us to let her

out of the restraints
run from the hospital
kill herself

She was smart; she was pretty. She was funny and artistically talented. What she could have been, would have been, might have accomplished were now hanging in the balance.

We talked. I watched, wondering over and over again whether she would ever be able to return from the edge. It was painful for me and for everyone else who worked with her.

While she slept and I alone watched her, my mind was in turmoil. She slept, at times so quietly she that looked like the child she never was, at times crying in her sleep, tormented by shadows trailing into her dreams. I watched hour after hour, day after day, as she seemed to improve and would then suddenly slip backward into an agony that we could neither fathom nor ease.

Dr. Carmichael and Maggie made plans to transfer her to another facility and then changed them. Plans were made for her to live out of state with relatives; those plans fell through, too. Child Protective Services couldn't allow her to return home and wouldn't place her outside her home. We couldn't release her because she had nowhere to go. Stacey was frustrated and confused; *we* were frustrated and confused.

The exit from the COU was a double door set up. Anyone leaving the unit needed a key to unlock the first door and enter a small anteroom. Only after the first door was closed and locked should the second door be unlocked to allow passage into the open corridor. The double doors provided an additional security measure to prevent unsafe patients from wandering or running away. In the event a patient somehow managed to get through the first door, the second door stopped them.

One afternoon Stacey had had an especially good day and had been out of restraints all day. As the afternoon wore on, though, she became agitated and talked more and more about wanting to

Deborah Clark Ebel, R.N.

leave. Nothing occupied her attention except her desire to get out of the hospital. We tried playing cards and we tried drawing. We tried reading and we tried talking. Nothing helped. Her dinner tray arrived, and after getting her situated, I told her that I was taking a break and would be back in half an hour.

I looked around to make sure that the way was clear before I put my key in the lock and turned it. I opened the door, and as I stepped through, Stacey suddenly appeared next to me in the ante-room.

She was breathing hard and fast. Excited and scared. "Debbi, *please*! I have to get out of here!"

"Stacey, *you can't* ..." I started, but I was interrupted by the sound of a key turning in the outer door lock. Someone was coming in, and Stacey could be gone in a flash! I yelled, "No!" and braced my foot against the door just as Stacey brushed past me and tugged at the outer doorknob.

She didn't pull hard. It struck me as more of a gesture than a legitimate attempt to run. We stood there, my hip jammed against the door and Stacey's hand gripping the doorknob. "Please," she whispered hoarsely, "I won't tell. Just let me go."

"I can't, Stacey, you know that. You need to be here to work all this through. I'm here because I care; I'm here to help." I shook my head, "It wouldn't help you to let you run away."

She looked long into my eyes and knew I wasn't going to move. Her hand dropped to her side, and she slowly walked to the inner door. "Will you let me back in?"

I unlocked the door.

*   *   *   *

Brittany was back. She had been brought in by the police during the night following a fight with her mother. She had been at Oak Haven several months previously and like many of those who returned, she thought she knew the ropes and could skate through. She didn't know it, but things were going to be different this time.

She whined. A lot. Sometimes it's almost easier to have a patient scream and swear and call me names than have them whine.

The Forgotten Future

"I need pajamas—" "My room is too cold—" "I need to use the phone—" "I need to sharpen my pencil—" "My room is too hot—" "I have a stomach ache—" With Brittany, it continued hour after hour, day after day.

She let us know straight out that she wasn't interested in doing any work while at Oak Haven because she didn't have a problem; she thought her mother did. The little I knew about her mother was that she probably *was* a good part of Brittany's problem, but learning to deal with it without trying to beat each other bloody was something that Brittany needed to work on.

The evening after her admission, she refused to eat dinner and came to the nurses' office complaining of another stomachache. She looked really uncomfortable, and I wondered whether something might really be wrong this time. I took a set of vitals and then put in a call to the medical doctor. He promised to see her before bedtime.

*   *   *   *

Spencer was another former patient who returned to us. Tall and actually rather funny-looking, he was the seventeen-year-old only child of an affluent local politician. He had been raised by his single-parent father after his mother moved to Europe to pursue her career as a photojournalist.

Spencer was different. His clothes were odd, his hairstyle was strange, and his favorite music was by a group called *They Might Be Giants*. Old re-runs of *Ren and Stimpy* were his choice in television. He was bright, even brilliant. He spoke in a soft and hesitant manner, and conversation with him could be a challenge. A lot of the other kids didn't understand anything he said. He was, in a word, *esoteric*.

He came to us after being expelled from his exclusive prep school. A lot of our kids had been suspended or expelled, usually for fighting or drugs, occasionally for theft. Not Spencer. He was expelled for hacking, a federal offense that carries a penalty of up to ten years. Spencer's dad and his lawyer were hoping Spencer would be tried as a juvenile, but they weren't very hopeful of that because Spencer would turn eighteen in three months and had been working with computers since he was six.

He and a friend had broken into their school's computer network and somehow managed to do a number of illegal operations. Not being fully conversant with computerese, I didn't understand exactly what he had pulled off, but I did understand that it had been serious. Very serious.

Spencer and his friend were picked up by federal marshals and, a mere four months from his high-school graduation, he was expelled.

He was depressed. It didn't seem to be the arrest and possible imprisonment as much as his feeling of having let people down.

His family

His school

Himself

He had come face-to-face with the understanding that no matter how smart and clever a person is, there's always someone smarter. He wasn't bitter or angry at the school or the feds. He acknowledged that he had committed a crime and said he would accept the responsibility and the consequences. He knew he had done something very wrong and very stupid.

What being caught did, though, was point out to him, in a very dramatic way, his vulnerability. Once he acknowledged his vulnerability in one area, past losses and missed opportunities hauntingly returned to remind him how he had covered up his feelings by intellectualizing his every word, every act, every thought.

Spencer was a good kid. He tried hard to keep his thoughts to himself and, having been so diligent about disguising his emotions, it took him a while to uncover his feelings.

When he first returned to us, he immediately set out to play his role.

"Jackie, do you have a minute? I want to show you something." Spencer usually preferred spending more time with staff than with his peers. Having been raised in a rather punctilious environment, he was more at ease with adults.

"Sure, Spencer." Jackie joined him at the table in the hall.

Spencer was excited. "Think of a number, any number. Okay,

now multiply it times two. Now, add eight."

I watched as Jackie performed the calculations in her head. I did the same in my own mind, with my own number.

"Divide that number by two and then subtract your original number. Okay. You got your number? Okay. Now correspond your number with a letter of the alphabet, like 'one' equals 'a', 'two' equals 'b', 'three' equals 'c', and so on."

"Okay, think of a country that starts with that letter. Got it?"

Jackie nodded. I had my country, too.

"Now move forward one letter in the alphabet and think of an animal that starts with that letter. Any animal, big or small. Now think of what color that animal is. Got it?"

We both nodded and waited.

"You're thinking of three things, right? A country? An animal? And a color?"

Nods all around.

Spencer smiled broadly. "That's impossible, Jackie. There are no gray elephants in Denmark!"

Jackie looked amazed, and I imagine I did, too. "How did you …" she began, and we all burst into laughter. A couple of the other kids wandered over and wanted to know what was going on and could they do it, too. Jackie and I moved away, still shaking our heads, so the kids could get together. Most of the jokes and card tricks and games that I knew had come from the kids. My problem was that I rarely remembered a joke beyond the next day. I had always envied those who could tell a joke or a story and tell it well. Comedy was not my forte.

*   *   *   *

Shortly before shift change, I looked up from my charting and saw Meghan striding up the hall toward the door, fully-clothed, carrying her coat and purse. Caitlyn reached over and casually flipped the switch that locked the swinging door. Without looking at us and completely unaware that we had secured the door, Meghan walked up and pushed against it. When it didn't give, she pushed again, harder, and then kicked the door. "Fuck!" she swore and whirled around to face me.

"Open the goddam door!" she screamed. "I want out of this fuckin' place."

"Meghan, you can't go anywhere tonight. C'mon. Let's go back to your room and talk."

"I ain't go-*in'* back to my room, and I ain't talkin' to you." She threw herself against the door full force. "Open it!"

We didn't seem to be making any progress. Bottom line was that she wanted to leave and we weren't going to let her.

Her demands became louder. Her abusive verbalizations devolved into threats.

A few members from the night shift arrived and were standing back at a discrete distance, watching to see how things would proceed. At first, I tried to get Meghan to walk with me back to her room in order to have a quieter place to talk where we wouldn't wake the other patients. As she continued to escalate, however, her room ceased to be an option because we couldn't allow her to become further out of control and stir up problems with other kids in the unit. She would have to spend the entire night in seclusion unless she was able to pull it together soon.

Caitlyn briefed the reinforcements. When she finished talking, they turned toward us and waited silently.

"Meghan, you can't leave, and you can't stay out here like this. You can either walk to the seclusion room with me, or these folks," I gestured toward the rest of the staff, "will help you. It's your choice. Make the right one."

"Nobody better not lay a fuckin' hand on me." Fists clinched and challenging, she still didn't comprehend that one way or another she was going to the seclusion room. She pounded on the locked door with her fists and gave it a final kick.

"Meghan ..."

"No! I told you I ain't *goin'!*" She then decided that I was the main obstacle to her leaving, and she angrily ran at me and shoved her full body into my left shoulder.

As staff members moved in and grabbed her, Meghan started to kick and punch wildly. As a group, we escorted her to the seclusion area where she was quickly moved onto the bed that had been wheeled into position. Despite the impossibility of escape, Meghan persisted in bucking and thrashing about, and we started applying thick leather restraint straps around each limb.

She was spitting, and I noticed that Eddie, the night nurse, was having trouble locking the restraint on her left arm. He was kneeling beside Meghan and had a huge blob of thick, white spittle rolling down his right cheek. He shifted his body slightly to remove himself as target and Meghan turned her head and spat right in my face.

My position at her shoulders was vital to keep her from banging her head, so I didn't have the option of moving away. One of the MHTs handed me a towel to place over Meghan's mouth to block her from spitting at me again, but I threw it to the floor. Placing towels over a patient's face was something I had seen at other facilities, but I didn't think it was safe. I didn't fancy the idea of being spat at again either, so, ingenuity being the mother of invention, I bent forward so that my long hair hung down between Meghan and me. I could hear her making hacking noises, and my hair grew damp from her continued spitting. It was disgusting, but to my way of thinking it was far less offensive than taking another hit directly in the face.

Once Meghan was safely restrained in the seclusion room and the night shift had assumed responsibility for her, I went to the staff bathroom to clean up. I pulled my hair back, secured it with a rubber band, and washed my hands and face. I felt dirty and couldn't wait to get home and take a shower.

Working conditions in mental health facilities have changed a lot in recent years, and from my perspective few of the changes are positive. Fewer staff are working with more and higher acuity patients. There is less administrative support personnel and fewer outside resources. More demands are being made of staff time and energy and while all these changes make things harder for the staff, the real losers are the patients. Some of these things played a part in Meghan's behavior that night; some had not. Her situation remained such that the only living option available for her at that time was a return to her mother's home. She thought living on the street would be a better deal.

By the next afternoon, Meghan was being discharged. She and her mother stood in glum silence as I explained discharge medications and follow-up treatment. They seemed completely uninterested in anything I had to say. Meghan had apparently decided that the most expedient way to escape from Oak Haven was to return to her mother's house. My guess was that she would be out of the house, maybe on the streets, maybe with a friend, within twenty-four hours.

After signing the discharge, her mother gave a clipped, "Thank you" and mother and daughter hurried toward the elevator. Meghan didn't think she had gotten anything out of her time with us, and I agreed. Like I always told the kids, *you get out of anything what you put into it.* I wondered where she would end up, where so many of the kids would end up.

*   *   *   *

At report the next afternoon we learned that it had been a reasonably good day. Stacey was still agitated, Spencer had become more withdrawn, and Brittany ...

"She's full of shit," reported Robin.

"We know that, Robin," I laughed. "Tell us something new."

Robin knew what our reaction would be and laughed along with us. "No, no, really. She *is* full of shit. They did an abdominal ultrasound today, and she has an impaction. She has to drink GoLYTELY to make her go. A whole two liters."

GoLYTELY is a liquid solution that is used to induce diarrhea. It tastes extremely salty, and even when mixed with fruit juice, most of the kids to whom I've given it say it's not very good. I've never found anyone who liked it, but it works. The patient has to drink a lot of it, typically four to eight ounces every fifteen minutes or so. Knowing Brittany's dislike of almost everything, I knew we were in for an unpleasant several hours.

"Has she started it yet?" I asked, hoping she had and was used to the taste by now.

"Nope. We decided to wait and let you do it." Robin grinned.

Brittany knew she was supposed to drink *something*, and when

The Forgotten Future

I went to her room at 4:00 with the first eight ounces, she was waiting for me. She took a sip and immediately spit it out. "I'm not drinking that stuff! No way!" She held out the Styrofoam cup, expecting me to take it.

"Brittany, did anyone explain to you why you have to drink this?"

"I don't care why. I'm not drinkin' it." She dropped the nearly-full cup into the trashcan with a thud and walked over and sat on the edge of her bed.

I decided to try the calm, rational approach, I explained to her about the impaction and how the GoLYTELY would make her "go". She didn't respond to that tact, so I explained the mechanical alternative, hoping to convince her of the benefits of GoLYTELY. That didn't work either.

By this time, her roommate had moved into action and whipped out a copy of the Patients' Rights information sheet. She vehemently pointed out Brittany's right to refuse medication.

I told Brittany again that this was her doctor's order and that it was important that she do what was ordered. Then I agreed with both girls that *yes, Brittany did indeed have every right to refuse medication, but that at the same time she also had to understand that there would be consequences to her refusal.*

"Like what?" she challenged, squinting at me.

"Like staying on the unit until you can do what is needed. Brittany, this is not for me; this is what is best for you."

She waited a few seconds and then said, "Okay. Let's go. To the seclusion room. I ain't drinkin' that stuff." Brittany walked out the door and headed down the hall. She looked back over her shoulder and beckoned to me. "C'*mon!*"

I followed her down the hall.

Ordinarily, I would have taken more time trying to convince a patient of the importance of following the prescribed regime, but in Brittany's case I knew that wouldn't work. She liked to be the center of attention and would take every opportunity to rally peer support for her position, that of poor-abused-patient-being-forced-to-drink-bilge-water. Also, I had seen the ultrasound report and knew it was absolutely imperative that she drink the GoLYTELY. I knew, too, she must have been awfully uncomfortable.

Placing her in the seclusion room removed her from her audience. She knew that as soon as she was taking the solution easily, without a lot of trouble, she could return to her room. Every fifteen minutes by the clock I offered her GoLYTELY. We tried it straight. We tried it over ice. We tried it diluted half-again with water. Eventually, we found the right combination: if we diluted it half-again with water, poured it over ice, and followed it with a full cup of ice water, she slowly and grudgingly would drink it.

"How much more?" she asked, pleased with herself after downing her first full cup.

I walked to the med room refrigerator and returned with the two-liter jug. I held it up for her to see.

"Shit!" she said and lifted her cup for a refill.

*   *   *   *

Word from the COU was that Stacey was becoming more stable, and it was hoped she could be discharged soon to her aunt and uncle in the Midwest. Her aunt was coming out to meet with Dr. Carmichael and Margie later in the week, and if everything worked out, Stacey would travel back with her aunt and be treated on an outpatient basis.

The crisis worker called to let us know that we had a new admission coming up. Jackie knew her from a previous admission and laughed about my admitting her.

Cyndy was seventeen, mildly retarded, and was in the manic phase of her bipolar disorder. She had been living with a friend from the Church of Scientology who had encouraged her to stop taking her medication. She had promptly flushed all of her lithium down the toilet and, soon after, became highly-agitated, sexually-inappropriate, wouldn't eat, and hadn't slept in days. When she arrived on the unit, accompanied by her Child Protective Services worker, she was wearing too much makeup and talking a mile-a-minute to everyone about everything.

After her worker left, I told Jackie I was taking Cyndy to her room to do the nursing admission questionnaire.

The Forgotten Future

"Good luck," Jackie smiled, smugly.

"Piece of cake," I replied.

Yeah. Right.

When I was in nursing school, I was intrigued when we entered our psychiatric nursing rotation. At first, of course, there was the typical over-identification by each student with whatever disorder we were studying at the moment. And then we were introduced to bipolar disorder, which was then known as manic-depression. As beginning nursing students, however, most of us didn't fully grasp the seriousness of the disease or its prevalence within the general population.

We learned that bipolar disorder is a serious, but treatable, disorder of the brain that is marked by extreme changes in mood, energy, thinking, and behavior, and that while in the manic phase, some sufferers do not eat, do not sleep, overwork, become hyper-sexual, and tend to have grandiose ideas about themselves and their abilities. The depressive phase is actually more common than the manic phase, however.

Until recently, a diagnosis of bipolar disorder was rarely made in childhood, but doctors can now recognize and treat the disorder in young children. The prevalence of young people diagnosed with bipolar has increased substantially in recent years, but it is unclear whether there is an actual increase in the number of young people with bipolar illness or whether it is simply over-diagnosed. Other disorders, such as attention-deficit hyperactivity disorder (ADHD), have symptoms similar to those of bipolar disorder and these may be mistaken for the latter.

I didn't know what to expect from Cyndy.

I sat at the desk in Cyndy's room and introduced myself and started to explain what we would be doing during the interview.

She interrupted and told me that she was glad to meet me, asked whether Debbi was my real name, said she once had a friend whose mother's name was Debbi, asked if I minded if she walked around the room while we talked, began rearranging the furniture, open and closed and then opened the window drapes again, asked me where I was born, told me where she was born, told me she liked boys, asked me if I liked boys, asked me if I liked her, and continued on without slowing down.

Every time I tried to return to the interview, she talked right over me. Finally, I gave up and decided to try again in a few days, maybe after she had been started back on lithium. In ten minutes' time, Cyndy had rearranged all the furniture in the room, made up her bed, opened and examined all the drawers and closets, checked out the bathroom, cleaned the sink and surrounding areas, and re-folded the bathroom linens.

I was exhausted.

*   *   *   *

The night had gone smoothly for a change. The kids were in bed and no one was acting-out. It was nice to think we could leave in less than an hour. I went into the staff kitchen to get some ice wa-ter, and when I returned to the nurses' office I found Ashley, the crisis worker, talking to Caitlyn. There was a tall, surly-looking teenage boy with them.

I sat down to continue my charting and at the same time half-listened to the conversation.

Jay, as I learned the young man was called, looked angry. Ash-ley looked like she couldn't wait to get away, and Caitlyn looked concerned. Jay was fourteen and had been abandoned by his par-ents three days previously at a nearby campground. New to the area, he had no relatives or friends to call for help and had been panhandling and shoplifting to keep himself going. A local shop-keeper called Child Protective Services when he noticed that Jay was still hanging out, and they, in turn, brought him to us.

Caitlyn asked Jay to sit down on the chair in the hall and then walked into the nurses' office. Jay continued to stand.

"What's this?" I asked Caitlyn. "An emergency admission?"

"No, can you believe it? They've known about this kid since 5:30 this afternoon and didn't bother to let us know. He's been downstairs for hours!" Caitlyn shook her head in disbelief. "They could at least have told us that he was coming so we could get a bed ready for him." She grabbed the IVAC thermometer and a blood pressure cuff and went out to escort Jay to his room.

The Forgotten Future

While Caitlyn was working with Jay, I finished charting and recorded the shift report. Twenty minutes later, Caitlyn returned to the nurses' office looking perplexed. "He's not saying much. I don't know if he's being oppositional or if he's just slow."

A couple of minutes later, Jay walked into the nurses' office and picked up his backpack without saying a word.

"Whoa," I said, jumping up and quickly walking toward Jay, "hold on. You can't take that 'til we go through it."

Every item brought onto one of Oak Haven's units had to be searched by the staff before a patient was allowed to have it. Cigarettes, matches, lighters, sharps of any kind, glass bottles, razors and mirrors, sometimes even shoelaces, were some of the items considered to be contraband, and weren't allowed. The kids usually complained about not being permitted to have their personal belongings, especially when they, themselves, weren't suicidal, but they didn't understand that prohibiting such items was for everyone's safety, not just for theirs.

"What do you need from your bag? I'll get it for you." I held out my hand to take the duffel bag, but Jay kept a tight grip on it without speaking. I stepped forward to take the bag, but Jay put it on the floor, unzipped it, and reached inside.

"I'll get it," I said as I hastily leaned over and reached into the bag myself. "You're not supposed to be here in the office."

Jay stopped, and our eyes locked, as a profound and unmistakable sensation of evil washed over me.

"I'm going to jail, you know," he said calmly.

"Oh, really?" I responded, holding out his toothbrush. I looked into his dark, angry eyes and shivered. "Is there anything else you need tonight? The night staff will go through the rest of your bag, and you can have it tomorrow."

He still stared coldly into my eyes and waited a beat before mumbling, "No." He took his toothbrush and sauntered down the hall to his room.

I turned to Caitlyn. "Oppositional," I said, but I couldn't shake the feeling of evil, unlike anything I had ever felt before.

Chapter 5
No Conscience

Someone rapped sharply on the COU window. I turned and saw Diana motioning to me from inside. I still had a few minutes before my shift started, and I walked to the window and leaned over to speak through the voice vent. "Hey! What's up?"

"It's Stacey. We're discharging her at 4:00. She wants to say good-bye."

I peered past Diana and saw Stacey in the COU community room, shifting from foot to foot, watching for my reaction to the news of her leaving. I smiled and waved and spoke through the grill. "Tell her I'll be back as soon as I get report. I want to say good-bye, too. Tell her I will definitely be back—and don't let her leave until I see her." Standing up straight, I made little hand motions to tell Stacey I was going to my unit and would return. She smiled and gave a little clap and a jump.

We had expected Stacey to be discharged soon, but we hadn't known exactly when. Stacey's maternal aunt lived several hundred miles away and had flown out to see how her niece was doing. She and her husband seemed genuinely concerned about Stacey and asked that she be allowed to come live with them.

All of the staff understood the significance of this very sincere offer, this reaching out to Stacey, and we were happy to see her leaving us with the opportunity to begin a new life. At the same time, however, there was great poignancy in her departure. We had grown used to her presence and her newly-emerging ability to laugh, the way she had plastered her artwork on the COU walls, her expressions of plans for her future.

Stacey had been with us for many months and we had become friends. We had been witness to her triumph over years of physical and sexual abuse and hidden psychological wounds caused by having been betrayed by someone she loved and trusted and on whom she had relied. Above all else, Stacey had survived. She had been to hell and returned—scarred, but stronger.

In recent days, she had shared her ambivalence about leaving, and we had talked about how sometimes people pass through our lives when we need them and how, even after they are gone, what we have learned from them—their impact on our lives and who we are—remains with us. Sometimes forever. Stacey's legacy to me would not be her survival; it would be her triumph. I believed her memories would be of triumph as well. That doesn't happen too often at Oak Haven. That kind of ending to a story is always, to us, a real bonus. It makes everything else survivable.

After I got report on my unit, I entered the COU and Stacey came running to give me a hug. We stood with our arms around each other, and she said excitedly, "I'm leaving in a few minutes. My Aunt Susan is in the business office signing papers." She paused and added, "I'm glad to be going, but I don't want to go, too. I'm scared … I'll miss everybody."

If we are fortunate, each of us will be touched during our lifetimes by a few very special people. For me, Stacey was one of those people. All that she expressed that I had given her—strength, courage, care and concern—I had also received from her. The opportunity to witness bravery and courage and determination beyond her years. The belief that maybe what I was doing really did make a difference.

Stacey's aunt arrived, and it was time for Stacey to leave. We embraced again, for the last time.

Tears streamed down her face. "I'll miss you, Debbi. I'll never forget you."

My eyes blurred, my throat ached. I gave her a quick kiss on top of her head and gently brushed a few damp strands of hair back from her eyes. She rested her head on my shoulder, still holding on like the world was ending. Or maybe it was just changing. We stood there for a long moment.

"I love you, Debbi," she murmured.

I gently broke our embrace and held her at arm's length. I paused before speaking, mulling over how best to respond. I wanted to tell her what was in my heart, but at the same time there was always that thin line between professional helper and friend. Do I speak what's in my heart, or would that be becoming over-involved and blurring the boundaries? This was a teenager—a young woman—about whom I cared so very much and whom I wished to have the life she deserved. Knowing that I would very likely never see her again, how did I want us to part?

It really wasn't a hard decision.

"I love you, too, Stacey. Don't ever forget how strong you are and how very special you are."

It was what was in my heart.

I like to think that she understood everything that I left unsaid, too. Then, with tears streaming, I turned and walked the length of the hall back to my unit. I couldn't look back.

*   *   *   *

Young people who are diagnosed with schizophrenia are particularly heartrending because it is an illness that affects every aspect of their lives for the rest of their lives. It can be treated with medication to help symptoms improve, but it is incurable. Many people don't understand the disease, or any mental illness for that matter, and they often react with fear, anger, or pity when meeting someone with, or hearing stories about, the illness. Much of the stigma aimed toward those with mental illnesses such as schizophrenia comes from media portrayals of those with the disease as out-of-control, unpredictable, violent, scary, dangerous, sad loners. In recent years, there have been major advances in treatment with the development of what are known as *atypical antipsychotics*, and these offer much hope to those suffering from these disorders as well as to their families.

Dylan had received a preliminary diagnosis of schizophrenia when he was sixteen. While he could have been maintained on medication outside of the hospital, he stopped taking the med because he didn't like the side effects. In the nine months that he had been on Zyprexa, a powerful antipsychotic drug, he had gained more than sixty pounds and didn't like his appearance. He reportedly was feeling better and had decided that he no longer required any medication.

Because he was doing so well and she was hoping against hope for a cure, his mother initially supported his decision to abruptly stop the med. Predictably, his condition deteriorated. He quickly became confused and paranoid and reported hearing voices. His behaviors and speech were bizarre, and he was almost compulsively sexual with partners of both sexes. He used a lot of marijuana and cocaine and believed the only effects the illegal drugs had on him were positive. In desperation, his mother finally brought him to Oak Haven.

Now seventeen, his career aspirations were to be a "free-lance computer-driven bounty hunter and FBI agent". The first time we met, he told me exactly that. I told him I wasn't exactly sure what a free-lance computer-driven bounty hunter and FBI agent did, so he spent about half an hour explaining it to me. I still didn't understand, but that's the way it was with a lot of our conversations. He was actually a very bright young man, and I enjoyed spending time with him, despite his frequently illogical and circuitous ramblings.

While Dylan was in Oak Haven, our goal was to restart him on medication and do some drug education and, of course, prevent his compulsive hyper-sexuality from being expressed on the unit.

*   *   *   *

Rachel approached me and asked in a hushed voice if she could speak with me. "It has to be in private. I don't want the other kids to hear."

With no idea what she wanted to speak to me about, I escorted her to Connie's office and closed the door behind us. "What's up, Rachel?"

"I know who has contraband on the unit, and I thought I better tell you."

I thought, *amazing*! Someone had finally listened to us when we talked about the dangers of bringing disallowed items on to the unit. "Okay," I said simply.

"Some of the kids have been smoking in their bathrooms. Meghan did, and I think Cyndy and Brittany, too. Brittany said Meghan gave her the cigarettes before she left." She hesitated, and added, "She offered me one, too, but I didn't take it."

"That's good, Rachel, because it's important that we keep things safe on the unit. Do you know if Cyndy and Brittany still have the cigarettes?" Meghan was gone, but if there were still cigarettes and matches or lighters on the unit, we could have problems. We would have to thoroughly search the rooms, which is something the kids never liked us to do.

"I don't know about Cyndy, but I do know that Brittany still has at least one cigarette in her room. It's in a little toothpaste box in her nightstand drawer. You won't say I told, will you?"

"No, I'm not going to tell, Rachel, but I'm glad you did. We have to be concerned about the safety of everybody on the unit. It's not a matter of being a tattletale or ratting on someone. If you knew about something dangerous on the unit and didn't tell us and then someone got hurt, I don't think you'd feel very good about things. It's a matter of acting responsibly." I rose to walk her to the door. "Is there anything else you wanted to talk about?"

"No. Just don't tell Brittany I told, okay?"

"No problem."

Howard was in the hall. "Want to give me a hand with a room search?" I asked as I walked by.

Quickly in step beside me, Howard asked, "Whose room?"

"Rachel says Brittany has a cigarette hidden in a toothpaste box in her nightstand. But she's afraid the kids will find out she told."

"Damn! I just gave Brittany a Level Two." Howard wasn't angry, just disappointed.

Many child and adolescent psychiatric units work with some

sort of level or other reward system. Kids achieve levels by actively participating in treatment and adhering to appropriate behavioral standards. The patients are rewarded for meeting these expectations by being awarded higher levels, and the levels, in turn, give the patients more privileges. These privileges may include things such as later bedtimes, wearing jewelry, increased phone time, leading select groups, and greater freedom on the unit.

Brittany had made progress since her bout with GoLYTELY. Although it had taken her a full day and a half to finish the two-liter jug of the liquid, it worked, and both her mood and her involvement in treatment had shown marked improvement. As a reward for her hard work and determination, Howard had given her a level increase with additional freedom and privileges—Brittany now had a half an hour later bedtime and an extra ten-minute phone call every day. The consequence for having contraband, such as the cigarettes, though, meant that her level would be dropped back to a Level One, and she would lose her newly-earned privileges.

"Guess she wasn't as ready as we thought," Howard sighed.

"Guess not." We reached room 413. I knocked gently and opened the door and peeked in. The girls were still dressed, so I opened the door wider and Howard and I both walked in.

"Ladies," I said, glancing around the room, "Howard and I are going to do a room search."

Brittany looked up from her desk and asked, "How come? I'm a Level Two. Howard just gave it to me."

Leisa rose from her bed and echoed, "Why?"

Covering for Rachel, I ad libbed. "Well, sometimes we do room searches when we give someone a Level Two just to make sure that the Level Two person is really ready for their new responsibilities and that everything's on the up and up." My eyes scanned the room. "Do either of you have anything in here that you shouldn't have?" I looked from Brittany to Leisa and back again.

Their response in tandem, "No, I don't have anything" followed by "go ahead and search" made me wonder for a brief moment if Rachel had deliberately misled me about the cigarettes as a set-up of Brittany. I had known kids to do that on more than one occasion.

The Forgotten Future

Howard searched the girls' bathroom and vents, while I checked the closets. I went through the piles of tangled clean and dirty clothes lying on the bottom of each girl's closet.

I stood on top of the desk to see if anything was stashed on top of either closet cabinet and found nothing except dust and a wadded-up piece of paper with "cocksucker" written on it. I tossed the paper into the trash and climbed down to check Brittany's bed. I turned back the bedding and lifted the mattress, feeling along the seams for any openings that might hold contraband.

Then, while Howard went through Leisa's nightstand, I took the items from Brittany's nightstand drawer and laid them out on top of the stand. A one-and-a-half ounce Colgate toothpaste box was among the collection, but I ignored it for the moment. Once the drawer was empty, I carefully examined each item and started putting things away. I picked up the toothpaste box and shook it, hoping I wouldn't find a cigarette. I was disappointed. Inside were two partially-smoked cigarettes and several matches.

I turned the box upside down and dumped the contents out onto the nightstand. "Howard, look at this."

Brittany sighed, "I'm sorry. I know I shouldn't have them."

Howard and I were both sorry, too, but she lost her Level Two and all the privileges that went with it.

*　　*　　*　　*

At 10:55 that night Howard and I sat in the nurses' office, completing the evening's charting and waiting for the night shift to arrive. Caitlyn was off the unit, taking a well-deserved break. We had been going full-out all shift and were exhausted. The constant up and down of our emotions was frequently more draining than any type of physical endeavor, so we took advantage of the few minutes of calm to talk about our hopes for Stacey, our concerns for Dylan, our frustration over Brittany and Cyndy and Jay and a myriad of other thoughts and feelings about other kids.

The harsh clang of the fire alarm broke through the quiet and demanded our attention. The rush of adrenaline I felt at the sound of the alarm carried me to the far end of the hall where I flung open the door to room 413, threw on the lights and yelled, "Get up! Go to the community room! It's a fire alarm! Up! Now!"

Brittany and Leisa were jolted out of their sleep. They jumped up and ran toward the community room as I moved on to the next room.

Howard was on the opposite side of the hall. He opened the door to 412 and was hit squarely in the face with released smoke and the musty spray of stale water from the sprinkler valves. I saw him reflexively take a step backward, out of surprise, horror, perhaps to gather a second breath. I knew that this was no drill; this was no false alarm.

Howard disappeared into the smoky wet darkness, and I quickly continued working my way up the hall, waking the kids and directing them to the community room. I thankfully noted that some of the night shift staff had arrived and were waking kids in the other rooms.

The smell. The worrisome mix of fire and water is an odor that, once experienced, is never forgotten.

Some months previously I had lost my home and most of my belongings in a fire. The smell clung to my hair and my skin, invaded my nose, my eyes, my throat. The smoke, the clamor of the fire alarm, the realization that much of what I had accumulated during my adult life was gone and that for all intents and purposes, my children and I were homeless, was inescapable.

For the next two months we stayed with various friends and relatives. We cried. We laughed. We discovered how insensitive some people can be and how genuine and caring others are. We mourned our loss; we rejoiced over what we had. Months later, though, upon picking up a book or other item rescued from the fire, the smell would hit hard and take me back to that night.

The hospital alarms continued to sound, and I reacted instinctively to shepherd the kids to the relative safety of the community room. I felt a dry tightness in my throat.

Clutching the check sheet, I called out each patient's name over the insistent alarm.

"Brittany!"

"Here!"

The Forgotten Future

"Lamont!"

"Yo!"

"Rachel!"

Silence.

"Rachel!"

"Here!" and so on until all except two were accounted for. Jay and Grant.

Howard had gone into Jay's room, room 412. The room with the smoke and the sprinkler. Was he still in there? And where was Grant?

I rushed to the door and yelled to the men and women in the hall, "I'm missing two! Jay and Grant. Jay is supposed to be in 412 where the fire is, and Grant is in 408. Howard went into room 412, and I haven't seen him come out. Everybody else is with me in the community room!"

I ran down the hall and saw the night nurse in room 408, trying to awaken a very sleepy Grant. Then I looked up and saw Jay and Howard coming up the hall, water dripping from their hair, their clothes soaking wet. Jay sprinted ahead of Howard and slipped into a seat just inside the community room door.

Everyone was accounted for.

Howard strode into the room, grabbed Jay's upper arm, and hauled him out of the chair and across the hall to the seclusion area. The kids hooted. I left Caitlyn in the community room with the kids and followed Howard. "What's ...?"

"He did it!" Howard responded angrily, jabbing his finger in Jay's direction. "I found him in the shower with the water running! *This little bastard started the goddam fire on purpose!"*

We stood outside the seclusion room, and Howard screamed at Jay to change from his clothes into pajamas. "Shoes. Clothes. Everything off!" Howard was angry.

I went to get pajamas from the linen room. As usual there were none. "Dammit," I muttered to myself and grabbed a couple of blankets and returned to the seclusion room. "There are no pajamas. You'll have to wrap up in these," I said holding the blankets out to Jay.

"Blankets? I ain't takin' off my clothes and wrappin' up in no blanket!" Jay seemed to think he had some choice in the matter.

He didn't.

"Everything off! Now! Before I take it off for you!" Howard demanded. He took a step toward Jay.

"Now!" I echoed the demand. We couldn't risk Jay still having matches or a lighter or whatever he had used to start the fire, and now certainly wasn't the time for a fashion statement. If all we had to offer Jay was blankets, then blankets it was.

Realizing that he had no choice, he started unbuttoning his shirt.

I crossed the hall and saw a dozen or so firefighters in the hall. The alarm continued to wail. A man clad in heavy firefighting gear who appeared to have some authority stopped and asked if I was the nurse in charge. After my affirmative response, he said things were under control and that we would have to talk at some point regarding building usage and possible criminal charges.

I wasn't in a position to make such decisions and told him he'd have to speak with one of the hospital administrators. He said he'd be around for a few hours and asked me to make sure that someone from the administration made contact with him.

I entered the community room. The mood was like a rowdy New Year's Eve party. Some of the kids were laughing and giggling and asking to have the kitchen opened to get something to eat. Some were grousing about having had to get out of bed. A few made fun of the firefighters laden with their heavy equipment. Some thought what Jay had done was funny and cool. On and on and on.

Just as I was about to speak my mind about the situation, Howard joined us. He slammed the door behind him and started to speak. Angrily.

He had barely begun when I cut across him. I was disappointed, and I told the kids so. Their inability to take the situation with any amount of seriousness, their insistence on turning the whole event into a joke … Their reactions epitomized what I had spent most of my career battling. Indifference. Lack of responsibility. Ignorance. Unconcern.

I told them that Jay had risked people's lives. *Their* lives. I reminded them that people die in fires, and that it's no joke. Staring Brittany straight in the eye, I hammered at the group that this was exactly why we didn't allow matches or lighters on the unit, that no one could ever predict what someone else might do. I told them I had lost my own home in a fire. I told them it was my job to keep them safe, and that the reason I was there was because I cared about them and what happened to them. Every single one of them. *Whether they wanted me to or not.* Then, blinded by tears of anger and disappointment, I turned and walked out the door. It was Howard's turn.

I never found out exactly what Howard said to them that night. I never asked, because it didn't matter. I said what I had to say, and Howard said what he had to say. I know he was mad as hell and that he let the kids know about it in no uncertain terms. I know that he was blunt and spoke to them in language that left no equivocation. He heard about that the very next day from an unhappy Director of Nursing.

I like to believe that the kids learned some important lessons that night. They were reminded that there are some people—and not always adults—who will put them at risk and never give it a second thought. Maybe they also learned a little something about responsibility and about people who care for them, asking nothing in return. All this came about in a way that, for many of them, probably made more of an impression and had greater impact than a hundred hours with a psychiatrist.

At home in the early morning hours, I dropped my coat and purse in the living room and walked directly through to the shower. I turned on the water as hot and as forcefully as I could stand. My eyes stung, my throat echoed a foul taste, and I had a cough. My hair smelled musty, as did my clothes, which went straight into the trash. As I stood under the hot spray, all I wanted was sleep. It didn't come.

At 3:00 the next afternoon, I exited the elevator on the fourth floor to the damp, acrid odor that clung to everything. The industrial fans placed throughout the length of the hall and in the six rooms at the far end of the hall hummed. Heavy-duty dehumidifiers gulped water from the waterlogged carpets, offering an occasional burp. Surprisingly, the wing wasn't condemned in any official sense, although the girls had been temporarily moved out and housed in the children's wing, and the boys were placed in rooms on the second floor.

The sleeping area of our wing would remain closed for at least two weeks while the carpets dried and the necessary repairs were made. The fire itself had been confined to a trashcan and caused no damage on our unit other than a few ashen tracks on the wall. Water damage from the sprinklers, however, was extensive.

The three floors below ours were flooded. Ceilings collapsed, walls peeled, and in the offices and classrooms on the first floor, books, cassette tapes, papers, and files had all been destroyed. With ceiling panels removed to allow the accumulated water to drain through, wires and insulation dangled loose. A heavy, musty odor hung in the air and accentuated the visual reminder of what might have happened to the entire hospital.

The Director of Nursing asked to speak to Howard privately. She looked serious. Howard and I exchanged glances before they left the room, and Robin started report with the mood of the unit.

For the most part the kids were coping well amid the confusion and changes around them. Some were angry about what Jay had done; some still thought it was a joke. Some couldn't have cared less.

A couple of them were angry and insulted over Howard's "lecture" and the fact that he had sworn and told them they had acted "stupid". Interestingly, some of the other kids had come to our defense and Robin added with a laugh, "they're calling you 'Mom' now. Howard is 'Bulldog'."

Oh god …

When Howard returned, he told me the DON had asked him exactly what he had said to the kids. He admitted that he had been upset and allowed that perhaps he might have chosen different words to express himself. The content of his message, however, was exactly what he had intended, and he refused to back down on that. Nevertheless, he gave the DON assurances that he would apologize to the kids during the evening's community meeting.

We entered the community room at 5:00 and were greeted with

smiles and calls of, "Hi Mom! Hi Bulldog!" Dylan called the meeting to order and asked if there were any staff issues to be addressed.

I began with an apology. I explained that the evening before had been a tense situation for everyone. I went on to tell the kids that Howard and I and everyone else who worked at Oak Haven were there to look after and keep them safe—every single one of them—and that we would do so in any way we had to in order to ensure their safety.

I told them that if I had done anything that in any way offended them, then I apologized, but I would not apologize for taking the situation seriously and acting quickly to do everything within my power to keep them safe. I would do exactly the same in the future.

"Bulldog" spoke next. He, too, reiterated that he was there to care for the kids. He apologized for his anger and his language and explained that when we couldn't find two of the kids, we had to consider, and be concerned about, all the possibilities. He told them that given the same situation, he would do it all over again.

What he didn't tell them, and what he had mentioned to me only briefly, was that many of the emotions and fears he had experienced that night were identical to those he had experienced many years before in a far-off country called Vietnam. Only then, the men he was searching for didn't make it. He hadn't wanted this outcome to be the same.

Dylan was next. Speaking to Howard and me, he said that a couple of the kids didn't understand and were angry. But then he said that most of them did understand that we had responded the way we had because we cared. That I had acted the way a mom who was worried about her kids would act. That I cared and wanted to make sure everyone was safe. *Mom.*

And *Bulldog.* Bulldog had been worried and wanted the kids to take the situation seriously. He cared about them and wanted them to be safe and learn from the experience. He had a job to do and wasn't going to let anything get in his way.

Dylan spoke lucidly and with real respect that evening. We had shown the kids we cared in a concrete and unequivocal way. Many of them had never experienced real caring before. Even before they stood and began to applaud, my eyes were already misting.

Deborah Clark Ebel, R.N.

A postscript worth mentioning: later that same evening the administration brought in pizza and soda for the third floor adult unit staff because they had had "a difficult and stressful evening" the night before. Those of us on the adolescent unit didn't even get so much as a "good job, guys, we wish you well".

But we didn't need to hear it from the administration. Two words—Mom and Bulldog—said it all. Nothing else was needed.

*   *   *   *

Jay remained locked in the seclusion room for many days. His meals were served on a tray and, although he was escorted to and from the bathroom, he was permitted to attend to his personal needs alone. He admitted that his intent had been to set the fire and escape down a back stairwell during the confusion caused by the fire alarm—he knew that whenever a fire alarm sounded, all the door locks automatically sprang open so no one would be trapped inside the building during a fire. He spent his time in the seclusion room sitting on a mat on the floor, staring at the door.

When we checked him each evening, we found him still sitting with eyes wide open and focused on the door. I got the sense that he was watching us. And waiting. If he spoke at all, he expressed himself in an arrogant and cold-hearted manner.

One afternoon, I arrived at work to find a note of "apology" that Jay had written to me at the insistence of one of my co-workers. The note was a single sentence in which he said that he hadn't intended to cause me any extra work. There was no remorse or concern about what he had caused to happen or what might have been the outcome, no apology for setting the fire itself.

For the most part, Jay sat and stared, and each day we wondered why he was still with us. Therapeutically, he was gaining nothing. Other than visits from Dr. Carmichael, Jay had no contact with anyone other than the nurses and MHTs attending to his needs. Why not a transfer to a state institution where they were better-equipped to handle such high-risk and criminally-oriented individuals?

While he remained back in the seclusion area, he had to be

watched closely, both on the monitor and in person. There were no additional staff assigned to our unit, so the staff we had was stretched even thinner than usual.

One afternoon, Dr. Carmichael gave Jay a written assignment intended to focus Jay's attention on his past behaviors and activities. He was told to write a two-page list of all the illegal behaviors he had ever engaged in.

Jay's response was a terse, written, "The only illegal behavior I had was turning on the sprinklers at Oak Haven. And a little bit of shoplifting. And I helped place a bomb in the World Trade Center and got away with it."

He wasn't delusional. He was incorrigible.

Dr. Carmichael returned the assignment to Jay and told him to specifically list, according to the age at which each incident took place, the number of times he had shoplifted, been involved in fights, burglarized someone's home, car or store, the number of times he had stolen something, the number of times he had started fires, and any other illegal activity that he could remember.

Jay tore the paper into tiny pieces and threw them into the hall.

We learned that the fire marshal was encouraging Oak Haven to file arson charges. Oak Haven's administration vacillated between "definitely" filing charges and rationalizing that "he's a psych patient who didn't have control over his actions. He needs to be understood".

While concerned for Jay, *my* understanding of the situation was that I had a unit full of other patients, not to mention the rest of the hospital that also needed to be protected. They were there for treatment they were not receiving because staff was busy putting out fires—no pun intended.

Jay's continued presence troubled and angered me. I had been at Oak Haven the night of the fire and I knew what could have happened. In my opinion, Jay knew exactly what he was doing and had done it with total disregard for the safety of anyone else. He had a history of setting fires, but never in a public place like this. Never in a hospital. If he were allowed to get away this time, it would be one more reinforcement that he could do anything he wanted without consequence.

Dr. Carmichael popped in to see Jay for a few minutes just about every afternoon. One day, after spending an especially short time with Jay, he rushed up to Howard in the nurses' office. "Do you have a key to the seclusion room?" he demanded.

Howard affirmed that he did, and Carmichael ordered, "Lock it. He needs to be locked." Carmichael abruptly walked away with no other comment, no explanation, no reason given. But, he appeared shaken.

What I couldn't understand and had trouble accepting was the way most in the administration appeared to be ignoring the seriousness of what had happened. People died in fires, and other than those who worked directly on the unit with patients, no one seemed to take the situation seriously. Up until this point, Oak Haven had a long-held policy that specifically excluded patients with a history of starting fires because of the inherent difficulty in monitoring them as well as the intensive, specific psychotherapy they required. Jay had proven to us what he was capable of, and there appeared to be no work being done on a treatment plan to meet his needs.

He had been abandoned by his parents, and that abandonment probably played a part in his subsequent behavior. But were we not now also abandoning him? We were providing no treatment for him whatsoever. He had serious problems, but as far as we could tell, the determinant of whether he stayed with us or was transferred somewhere else more appropriate seemed to be that every day we carried Jay on our books meant an additional day of billable services. Therefore, he remained in our seclusion room.

And watched our every move.

One evening a staff member discovered that Jay had secreted several pieces of plastic tableware provided on his meal tray, breaking them into sharp points and hiding them inside a slit in his floor mat. After that he was served only finger foods. No tableware allowed.

We learned that Dr. Carmichael planned to return Jay to the open unit. Howard and I were particularly concerned about this, but there was nothing we could do. Fortunately, several days before Jay's planned repatriation to the open unit, things were taken out of our hands.

Just before the day shift left for the evening, I went to check on Jay and found him in the hallway, arguing with Robin and about to exit the area. He had been pounding on the unlocked heavy metal door, demanding an early dinner, and he got tired of waiting.

Robin was insisting that Jay return to the seclusion room, but he refused, and it was obvious that a standoff was taking place. When I arrived and told him to go into the seclusion room, he stared into my eyes for a long time. A very long time.

Slowly, without taking his eyes from mine, he walked into the seclusion room and pulled the door shut behind him.

I locked it.

When Jay wanted to go to the bathroom later that evening, my gut told me I shouldn't be alone in the transfer. Howard was my backup.

I unlocked the door, and Howard escorted Jay, clad in green two-piece hospital-issue pajamas, across the hall to the bathroom. While Jay was out of the seclusion room, I took the opportunity to do a quick search to make sure nothing had been hidden away. I checked the heater vent, the windowsill, and the mat. All clean. I looked up at the camera mounting, and everything was as it should be. Then, I waited outside the bathroom door with Howard.

Jay emerged from the bathroom and padded back across the hall to re-enter the seclusion room.

"All set?" asked Howard.

Jay had taken a long time in the bathroom, and both Howard and I really needed to get back out to the rest of the kids. For a brief moment, I was tempted to just forgo searching Jay and allow him to return to the seclusion room. I decided to check him anyway.

I stepped in front of Jay, just as Howard said, "Hold up, there. We have to search you."

Jay mumbled, "Nobody else ever searches me." That was part of my and Howard's frustration. We were probably more suspicious of Jay than the rest of the staff because we had seen him in action and neither of us trusted him one iota.

Howard started to pat down Jay and then told him to lean against the wall, palms flat. Jay spread his legs and leaned. I noticed his right hand was partially closed, his knuckles white.

"Flat," I said. "Your hand needs to be flat against the wall."

He grunted and slowly straightened out three fingers. Something was wrong …

"Howard, wait! Check his hand." Instinctively, I took a step backward to put some space between us. "Jay, what's in your hand?"

The scene unraveled in slow motion, as Jay glowered at me over his right shoulder and flexed his hand to show an eight-inch steel metal rod. He turned sharply and made a sudden move toward me. Then, he abruptly stopped. He coolly turned the rod over in his hand and backhanded it to me.

"Take off your shirt!" said Howard.

"I don't have nothin' else," scowled Jay.

"You wouldn't tell us if you did! Now, take it off!"

Jay, how did you think you could get away with this?" I asked, holding the rod a safe distance from him.

"I didn't think you'd search me. Nobody else ever does."

Jay took off his shirt and his socks, loosened the elastic around his waist and shook. Howard patted him down again. Clean.

He walked into the seclusion room, and we locked the door behind him.

The steel rod was part of the drain mechanism from the bathroom sink. Jay had unscrewed it and palmed it—who knows what he had planned? But I shuddered to think of what he might have done if we hadn't discovered it.

I notified Dr. Carmichael about what had happened and requested a renewal order for locked seclusion. We usually had problems getting his cooperation, but this time he went along with my recommendation and ordered, *"locked seclusion for up to twelve hours for patient and others' safety. Order not to be discontinued until after Dr. Carmichael has seen the patient."*

At report the next day, I learned that Jay was being transferred to a state facility at 4:00. He didn't know it yet, but the State Police were already on their way to pick him up. At precisely 3:55, the receptionist called to say the officers had arrived and were waiting in the lobby.

We called for additional staff, hoping to avoid a struggle with a show of force. We fully expected Jay to angrily act out when he learned of the transfer, but that didn't happen. He remained calm, and the MHTs accompanied Jay to the first floor where he was unceremoniously cuffed and shackled for transport to the state juvenile detention facility some thirty miles away.

That was it. No struggle. No resistance. As suddenly and as quietly as he had arrived, he was now gone.

With his departure, Jay took much of the tension and uncertainty off the unit. What he left behind, however, was a question in the minds of many as to whether or not we were doing our absolute best for every child in our care.

*   *   *   *

Kelly was sixteen and beautiful. Model thin, with high cheekbones accentuating her very patrician nose, she frequently tossed her cropped brown hair and flashed a brilliant smile. Especially when there were males around. *Teenage* males, that is.

She came to Oak Haven following a suicide attempt in which she swallowed a significant number of over-the-counter sleeping pills and received treatment with charcoal and lavage at a local emergency room. She admitted to some minor drug use, and her history included a single incident of an adult male taking nude photos of her when she was twelve years old. She denied any other sexual or physical abuse. In the weeks just prior to the suicide attempt, she had been staying up all night and sleeping all day.

Whenever she was in a group, she put a lot of energy into encouraging, albeit subtly, negative behavior among her peers. The boys liked to posture and show their tough-guy exteriors, and she was an appreciative audience.

She giggled.

Both boys and girls liked to toss out sexual innuendoes and frequently overtly sexual comments about their prowess, their experiences, about their or another's anatomy.

She giggled.

She toted around magazines such as *Vogue, Cosmo, Self, Muscle and Fitness,* all of which showed partially-clad and sexually-provocative young women and featured articles such as *Give Him a Sexual Night He'll Remember.* Kelly enjoyed sharing these with the other kids, especially the boys.

And, of course, she coyly giggled.

Given the superficiality with which she presented herself, I was surprised, and more than a little skeptical when, during our first lengthy one-to-one, she began to disclose what her life was really like.

Her mother had had eight "serious" relationships since divorcing Kelly's father twelve years previously. Kelly had a younger brother and sister, and all three of them had a different father. She talked about her need for a mother who showed some interest, some involvement, in her life.

"Like, for my Christmas concert at school. I wanted her to come, but she stayed home, drinking and waiting for a phone call from her boyfriend. All the other kids' parents were there and I felt funny because my mom wasn't there."

She had grown up without a nurturing parent to instill any sense of self worth, any sense of who she was or what she wanted to become. Her mother's concept of self was a reflection of others' opinions of her and, just as children imitate the roles modeled by their parents, Kelly's sense of self was based on how others reacted to, approved of, sought after her. She had no inward balance, no awareness of who she was or what she wanted. She presented herself and behaved in a way to please others and receive their approval.

She didn't like that in herself.

She spoke at length about her mother's emphasis on appearances. Cosmetic surgery. Clothes. Fashion. Image. How things *looked.*

And about the reality. Never enough food in the house. About staying home from school to baby-sit for her brother and sister while their mother slept. About how her seven-year-old sister had gone to a neighbor's house to ask for something to eat. About how her four-year-old brother had once "shit" in a neighbor's backyard because their mother was asleep and the house was locked and he had to go to the bathroom. "He didn't shit in our yard because he knew mom would get mad. I went over and cleaned it up out of their yard. It was embarrassing."

After our talk, I understood her a little better. She was suffering and covered it all up for the rest of the world. She smiled and put everyone at ease.

Then she went back out on the unit and started flirting and giggling again.

*   *   *   *

Thirteen-year-old Abram stood at the door to the nurses' office, He had been admitted during the day shift and was asking his zillionth question about what was required in his autobiography. His pants sagged to a point just north of indecency and he swayed from side to side as he spoke. He was dirty. And smelly. His shoulder-length hair hung in grimy strands that he controlled with frequent tosses of his head.

Caitlyn answered the questions to his apparent satisfaction, and he returned to his room. A few minutes later, he was back at the nurses' office door. His attitude was no better than his hygiene. "Man, why do I have to do all this work? This place is fucked!"

His dad and stepmother had brought him to Oak Haven because of Abram's recent sexual inappropriateness. Point-blank, he had taken to exposing himself to his twenty-three-year-old stepmother, watching her dress, undress, and bathe, and masturbating whenever and wherever he felt like it.

We also learned that the family liked to smoke together. Not tobacco. Marijuana. A complicating factor.

Several days prior to admission, his stepmother had found Abram masturbating on the couch in the living room. After she confronted Abram and asked that he do that in his own room, he went over and brushed up against her and grabbed her breast. His father called Abram on his behavior, and Abram began making threats of suicide.

Throughout his stay with us, Abram questioned and challenged every single thing he was told to do, and he usually did so with language that was hostile and threatening and intended to degrade its target. He was tough and he was angry. He was another kid who despite his small stature, I wouldn't trust for a second.

* * * *

Brittany had changed a lot. She had transformed into a mature young woman right before our eyes.

She had been different since the night of the fire. She had become noticeably more serious and responsible about changes she needed to make in her attitude and behavior. She had begun to really work on her issues with her mom, even though her mom wasn't ready to make the same kind of commitment. Brittany had resolved to be part of the solution, not part of the problem.

She appeared to accept who her mom was: an exotic dancer, a substance abuser, a mother who wasn't interested in being a parent. Brittany didn't understand or like it, but she accepted it. It was reality. In many ways she had become far more mature than her mother.

When her mother came for family therapy dressed in a white silk suit cut-down-to-there, Brittany's quiet maturity allowed her to refrain from making any comment. The social worker did, though, and asked that the next time she dress a little more conservatively since the teenage boys' tongues were hanging out and dragging on the floor.

When her mother visited and made comments about Brittany never amounting to anything, Brittany's new sense of self prevented her from being baited. Brittany called me at work several months after discharge to proudly announce that she was on the honor roll—"for the first time in my life!"—and that she was considering the possibility of college.

It was also her new confidence after discharge that allowed Brittany to survive numerous verbal and physical fights with her mother and which allowed her to call the unit and discuss options for staying safe until the crisis passed.

The Forgotten Future

Both before and after her discharge, Brittany and I talked frequently about how she had changed. I told her she was a brat when she first came to Oak Haven. She laughed, cocked her head to one side and answered, "Yes! I was! I *was!*" She was proud of her progress, and I was honored to have been a part of her life.

She had no support at home and only limited support from her father and an aunt. But she had tried and she was doing her best and that's all anyone needs to do.

*   *   *   *

Taylor was sitting in bed talking with her roommate when I checked on them during rounds. It was close to lights-out, but they still had a few minutes. Taylor had moved her bed so that it was tucked nicely into a corner of the room, and she sat with several pillows propped up behind her. Her roommate only had one pillow. A squashed, flat plastic one like you find in most hospitals.

Taylor was somewhat self-centered. Vain. Narcissistic. She really believed the world was her oyster. She had been transferred to Oak Haven after being caught having intercourse with a teenage boy at another hospital and the administration there felt they could no longer manage her.

She had two stories she loved to tell. The first was that eight months previously she had given birth to a beautiful baby boy who had been taken away and given to her cousin to raise. She had everyone convinced of the truth of this story until we discovered a couple of reports from recent ob-gyn exams indicating that she had never been pregnant.

Her other favorite story was that she was an American Indian princess. The exact tribal affiliation was vague, but, who knows? She *looked* like she might be Native American, with her long beautiful black hair, and she certainly had a haughty, princess-like air.

"Oh, hi, Debbi. I hoped you were Howard." She leaned back into the pillows, looking somewhat disappointed.

As usual, my eyes scanned the room for anything out of place, or unusual, or strange in any way, but everything seemed to be okay. "He's down at the office. Did you need to talk to him or will I do?" I leaned against the closet door, my ankles crossed, and waited.

"No, I just thought maybe he'd be doin' rounds tonight."

"Nope, not tonight. Just me." I straightened and headed toward the door.

"Debbi?" Taylor said, giggling. "I got a question."

I paused and turned away from the door. "What's up?"

"I think Howard's hot. I mean, for an older guy. I mean, I think he's sexy and I wouldn't mind fucking him." More giggles.

Oh god. Oh shit. Please don't say this, Taylor.

There had been several good looking, just-out-of college male mental health techs at the hospital where I had previously worked. They were eager and enthusiastic, challenged by the kids' problems, and easily flattered by the attention paid them by some of the adolescent female patients. The nursing staff repeatedly reminded the MHTs to never go into a female patient's room alone with the door shut and, if at all possible, to stay by the open door to do their talking. The risk of a false accusation by an angry or rejected young woman was too high.

Fortunately, they took our advice, and we never had that problem. Howard, however, had been in this line of work for a long time and had no hesitation about going in and doing one-to-ones behind closed doors with any of the kids, boys *or* girls. He seemed to think and act as if he were immune to such problems, although he once did show me a poem from a seventeen-year-old girl and asked me what I thought of it.

"You have a problem," I said, handing the paper back.

"I thought so," he replied as he folded the paper and put it into his shirt pocket. "I just wanted to know if you thought it was the same kind of poem I thought it was."

"It is," I confirmed. Enough said.

That time Howard talked to the girl and explained his role and his relationship to all the patients and very clearly let her know he wasn't interested. End of problem.

This one worried me though, so when I got back to the nurses' office, I reminded Howard to never, ever, put himself in the position of being alone with Taylor. I told him what she had said and he let out a long, slow whistle.

The Forgotten Future

During the rest of Taylor's hospital stay, she tried to get close to Howard as often as she could. He managed to avoid any close contact with her, though, so there were no problems.

Nevertheless, he seemed relieved when she was discharged. I certainly was.

*   *   *   *

The girl lying motionless in the bed was bruised and battered. Her swollen and discolored face looked painful, and I stood and stared for a couple of minutes. A purple-turning-black bruise covered the entire right side of her face. Dried blood crusted her lower lip and fresh blood oozed from several small cuts beside and below her nose.

I called her name and lightly touched her shoulder to let her know I was there to take a set of vitals: temp, pulse, respiration, and blood pressure. She murmured her assent, but didn't open her eyes.

Her vital signs were all elevated, which was to be expected. "Crystale, hon, I need to ask you some questions, okay?"

"Uh huh." She shifted slightly, making an "uhhhh …" sound as she moved.

"Crystale, do you know where you are?"

"Nnnnh …" She sounded groggy. "At th' hospital. Mmmm … Tall Tree Hospital."

"Close enough." Oaks were trees. "Okay, what day is it?"

"Oh, shit. Sunday? No. Saturday, I think."

"Good. It's Saturday afternoon. Okay, last one. Who's the President?"

"Hillary Obama." Long pause, then she opened one eye and said, "That's a joke, ya know? I know it's still President Bush. So, now you know my brain's all right. Can I go back to sleep?"

"In a couple of minutes. How are you feeling?"

"Like shit. Can I get some Tylenol?"

"I'll bring it down. How about some ice? For your face?"

"Yeah, okay."

I left to get the Tylenol and ice, reviewing in my mind what I knew about Crystale. She was fourteen and lived on the streets. She was also a gang member and made her living as a prostitute. She had been at Oak Haven twice before, and all the staff knew her. This time she had been found unconscious on the sidewalk outside a convenience store, badly beaten by fists, a brick, and a pipe. The police took her to the emergency room, and once she was medically cleared, she was transferred over to us.

She had been beaten by sister gang members who believed she was trying to steal the affections of their pimp. It was a very complicated scenario, and I had to work hard to keep the players straight. Bottom line, she had been hurt badly and was lucky to be alive.

I returned to Crystale's bedside with Tylenol, water, an ice pack, and our Polaroid camera. "Here ya go, Crystale. Can you sit up to take this?"

Moving slowly and resisting any help from me, she sat up and downed two white pills and a full glass of water. I explained that I needed to take some pictures to show what her injuries looked like, and she gave her permission. I took the whole roll. Her face, the inside of her mouth, the back of her head, her legs, her abdomen, and her back. She was a mess.

"Why don't you lie back down and get some rest. I'll bring your dinner when it comes."

She managed a weak smile and whispered, "thanks", then laid back and pulled the covers up to her chin.

I think she was asleep before I even reached the door.

Chapter 6
Baby Blues

Kelly leaned out her door as I approached. She was chewing her thumbnail. "Debbi? Can we talk?"

She had managed to avoid me for most of the shift, and now it was half an hour past bedtime. I hesitated, but before I could answer, she added, "It's really important."

Many times the staff would be so involved with other assignments that the kids would get a response like, "Just as soon as I finish up here" or "I'll be there in a couple of minutes" and then fail to get back to the patient. That wasn't a problem if what was involved was something trivial or something the kids could take care of themselves. On the other hand, putting off someone who had something important to discuss might have the effect of turning them off completely and they might never ask to talk to any of us again.

So my deal with the kids was that if they needed me to tell me straight out that it was important. That's why I was there. I motioned Kelly out of her room and asked where she wanted to go to talk. Would the community room be okay? All the other kids were in bed, so we would have privacy there.

She sat in one of the upholstered chairs facing me and began by telling me she didn't know how to begin. We talked, and eventually she told me that she had lied to the drug ed group about the extent of her drug use and wanted to know how she could go back now and tell them what and how much she had really been using. She said she had lied to the group because she didn't want to look bad.

Kelly talked about drinking and smoking pot every day. She sounded throaty and told me she had tried cocaine on several occasions. She took caffeine pills to stay awake at night and then took Benadryl to sleep during the day. Almost as an afterthought, she mentioned having used LSD three times. "I didn't like what happened," she said, looking away.

"Tell me," I said. I had a hunch there was more to this than guilt over lying to the drug ed group.

"I had flashbacks," she said, softly. She scratched the back of her left hand with her right thumb, and then studied it. "Flashbacks about the man who took pictures of me." She looked up. "Dr. Evans says I have to talk about it, but it's hard to talk about things like that with him. I don't like older men, and I don't trust them either. I get real scared when I have to sit in a room alone with him."

Kelly told me about the flashbacks that began the first time she used LSD. She started having recurrent nightmares about the man and the pictures, and that was when she started staying awake all night and sleeping during the day. "I only have nightmares if I sleep at night. If I sleep during the day, I'm okay."

She continued talking, explaining how her drug use had increased and how it had affected the way she lived. I asked questions when something wasn't clear, but once she started, she didn't need much encouragement. She told me about the nightmares and how they made her feel. Then quietly, and with great concentration, she told me about a day when she was twelve.

"I was walking along the railroad tracks behind my neighborhood, and there was this guy working on his bike. He called me over. He said 'C'mere. I won't hurt you.'"

"And you went over?"

"Yeah. I didn't want him to think I didn't like him or somethin'. He looked regular and he said he wanted to take some pictures of me and that he wouldn't hurt me." She sighed and looked up at the ceiling. She was remembering that day, and I sat listening to the silence.

She picked at her thumb's cuticle and then looked at me and picked some more. She took a deep breath and continued. "He told me to sit down with the railroad tracks running between my legs and pull up my shirt. Then he told me to drop my bra. I did what he said, and he took some pictures—Polaroid ones—and showed them to me. I didn't want to look, but I did."

"Then he told me to pull down my pants and he made me reach down and pull myself wide open so he could take some more pictures. He made me touch and rub myself and put my finger inside. I thought it was sick, but I kept doing it. I knew I should run away, but I was scared he'd grab me and kill me. He kept taking pictures, and then he took his thing out and started rubbing it 'til he came." She looked anguished at the recollection. "Finally, he just left. I felt dirty, and I was really disgusted about what I did with my hands. I wanted to get the feeling off, so I rubbed and rubbed my hands on the wood railroad tie. I kept rubbing 'til they had all these splinters and were bleeding." She looked at her hands and rubbed them together.

"When I got home, I took a shower and scrubbed myself all over. I felt so dirty and my hands hurt from the splinters." Her eyes narrowed and she sounded angry. "You know, those pictures are still out there somewhere. He still has them. Sometimes in my nightmares, I go on the Internet and my picture is there with a message that says 'Do you know who I am? C'mon guys, do me,' or something like that. I'm afraid he'll come looking for me; that's why I dyed my hair. Back then it was long and blond." She reached up and ran her fingers through her cropped brown hair.

"Every time I did LSD it was like it was happening all over again. And even when it made me feel horrible to go through it all again, I wanted to. Just to prove to myself that it really did happen, that I didn't imagine it and that it wasn't my fault. Now I'm afraid that I'll go back and use more and more just to know it really happened. Is that sick?"

We talked for a while longer and Kelly described how her memories frightened her, but at the same time she felt inexorably drawn to relive the experience in order to "prove" it happened. It was a troubling tale, yet what bothered me deep down inside even more than Kelly's story was that it didn't shock me. It didn't have the impact on me that it should have. I had heard too many similar stories, too many times, for too long.

That saddened me.

*   *   *   *

The fire alarm sounded just before 10:00 Tuesday evening. I jumped from my chair in the nurses' office, ran to the end of the hall, and threw open the door to room 415.

"Get up," I shouted. "Go to the community room! Now!" The girls jumped up from their beds and hurried down the hall, no questions asked.

Howard was on the other side of the hall, rousting kids from their somnolent state. For the most part, they responded quickly, with only a few complaints about being awakened. In room 411, Kelly sat on the edge of her bed, slowly and deliberately putting on her shoes and tying them.

"Kelly, out! Now! You have to go to the community room. It's the fire alarm!"

She complained loudly about having to get up and let me know graphically that she thought both the situation, and I, were profoundly stupid.

"Move! Now! Move!" I sounded like a drill sergeant, but the kids were my responsibility, and after the previous month's fire, I wasn't taking any chances.

Kelly strolled down the hall like she was on a spring walk along Park Avenue. I moved on to the next room, and then the next.

I threw open Abram's door and was taken by surprise. The faint smell of smoke and sputtering sprinkler system told me we were in for it again. Suddenly, I was thrown against the wall, full force, right hand slammed hard against the metal doorjamb, right hip clipping the wall.

"Fuck you, bitch!" he screamed. "Fuck you!"

Abram was out of control, cursing and yelling, and coming

straight at me. Suddenly, out of nowhere, Howard appeared and grabbed Abram in a giant bear hug. Regaining my balance, I caught a glimpse of kids hurrying down the hall to the safety of the community room. The alarm continued to wail.

Abram struggled as Howard half-carried, half-pulled, half-dragged him to the seclusion room. I ran past them to the community room and thrust the census board into Caitlyn's hands. "Count 'em!" I shouted and rushed ahead of Howard to open the seclusion room door. I could see the kids standing in the community room, talking and giggling. It was just a big joke to them. My head began to throb.

"I'm gonna kick your ass! I'm gonna fuck everybody! I'm glad your wife is dead! You didn't deserve her! You probably killed her. Yeah, you probably beat her to death! I'm gonna get a gun and come back here and kill you!" Abram continued fighting and screaming at Howard, his face contorted with rage. "I didn't do nothin', you fucker!"

Howard shoved Abram into the seclusion room and assumed a stance that dared Abram to come at him. Abram glared back, but he didn't move.

In the back of my mind I was thinking about the sixteen other kids in the community room with Caitlyn. Although things seemed to be under control, I worried that one of the kids might try to take advantage of the confusion. I needed to get back out there with them.

We didn't know what Abram had used to set off the alarm and sprinkler, and we had to make sure he didn't still have matches or a lighter on him. I grabbed a pair of hospital pajamas from the shelf and tossed them toward Howard. "He needs to change."

Howard took them and started toward Abram. The alarm fell silent.

"I ain't puttin' on no pajamas," Abram began. Howard clutched the green hospital pajamas and walked into the seclusion room. The door slammed shut behind him. He was pissed. I turned and walked out to assess the rest of the situation.

I met Randall, one of Oak Haven's maintenance workers, in the hall. He told me we were lucky this time. Abram had set fire to a few pages from his notebook and had waved them overhead to set off the sprinkler. Fortunately, the sprinkler quickly put out the small blaze so there wasn't any real smoke or flame damage and this time the sprinkler had been turned off before any serious water damage had been done.

Caitlyn was in the community room comforting our very frightened new admission, Marilyn. *Welcome to Oak Haven, Marilyn.* Her eyes were wide, and she looked scared to death.

Some of the rest of the kids had raided the patients' kitchen and were happily munching away on the few packages of crackers and containers of juice they could find. A few of the kids turned and excitedly asked, "How come Abram's in the seclusion room?" "What happened?" The others couldn't have cared less. It was party time.

Later, Howard walked into the nurses' office and threw Abram's clothes and watch down on the desk. He jabbed his finger toward the seclusion room and growled, "That mother-fucker can stay back there ''til he's discharged. He doesn't give a shit what he does or who he hurts."

Howard's face was red and contorted, and his eyes were damp. I realized he was fighting back tears. His wife had died suddenly and tragically a couple of years previously, and when Abram started in on Howard's deceased wife, he had slammed hard where it hurt. As much as it can humanize us to the kids to tell them about things we have experienced and survived, it exposes us to attack when they want to get back at us. And since we're all human, someone honing in on our vulnerabilities shoots us in the knees.

By now Caitlyn was herding the kids back to their rooms, and Randall was cleaning up in Abram's room.

"Do you want to take a break?" I asked Howard. "Take a walk; go have a cigarette ...?"

"Yeah, I need a break. I really need a break. This is bullshit." Howard ran his fingers slowly through his hair and walked toward the elevators.

I knew he wasn't just talking about tonight. We—the adolescent unit staff—were all coming to the realization that with the insurance-driven shortened hospital stays and less than optimal staffing, the teenagers in our care were being deprived of treatment they desperately needed. Because of heavy case loads, the clinical staff was unable to devote adequate time to much-needed therapy, and with the usual practice of having only one registered nurse on each shift, no matter the number of kids on the unit, the kids were not receiving adequate care from the nurses, either. Hospital and outside resources had been greatly curtailed, and, as a result, our patients had too much downtime doing things such as watching movies or sitting in their rooms alone.

As a result, seeing significant change in any of our kids was becoming rare. Even more troubling, however, was our awareness that because of the frequently inadequate staffing, people's safety, perhaps even their lives, were at risk.

I put in a call to Dr. Carmichael's service to get an order for locked seclusion. Twenty-five minutes later he returned my call. I hated talking to him. He could be rude or condescending, depending on his mood.

Shortly after I started working at Oak Haven, I had called Dr. Carmichael late at night for an order, and he went absolutely berserk on the phone. I was stunned because I wasn't used to dealing with such a prima donna. My co-workers told me that that was his style and not to worry about it. Twenty minutes later, he called back to apologize, but it was a backward sort of apology in which he told me what a tough night he was having. That he had a patient who was suicidal. That he was tired.

I was tired, too. *Everybody* was tired.

I accepted his apology and thanked him for calling back, but I didn't tell him it was okay. It wasn't. Since then my exchanges with him had been brief and formal. Not unfriendly. Just to the point.

"Dr. Carmichael, Abram started a small fire in his room and set off the sprinklers. I'd like an order for locked seclusion for the night."

"Well, why'd he do that?" Carmichael's nasal whine irritated me more than usual.

"I don't know, but he did. And when we took him back to the seclusion room, he was out of control and threatening staff." What

Deborah Clark Ebel, R.N.

I really wanted to say was *how the hell do I know why he did it? You're the psychiatrist.* I refrained. "So I need an order for locked seclusion."

"Is he still out of control? Do you really think he needs to be in restraints?"

"Not restraints, Dr. Carmichael. We just need the door locked. Right now he's pounding on the door and continuing to threaten staff, and a staff member has to hold the door to keep him from coming out."

"Four hours," he said tersely. "You can lock him for up to four hours, to be processed out at the R.N.'s discretion."

"Dr. Carmichael, we need twelve hours to get him through the night shift. It's almost 11:00 now, and there are only five staff for both the children's and adolescent units tonight. They just aren't staffed to keep him back there unlocked. It's not safe. For anyone."

He was silent.

Finally, and abruptly, he directed, "Twelve hours. I'll see him in the morning. Don't let him out until I have a chance to assess him. Do you need anything else?"

"No, Dr. Carmichael. Thanks for the order."

He hung up without replying.

*　　*　　*　　*

Sarah was shy, quiet, and two months pregnant. Only thirteen, she was pregnant for the second time, having suffered a miscarriage a year earlier. She was in Oak Haven because her current pregnancy was causing serious problems within her family. Her grandmother wanted her to have an abortion. Her mother forbade her to have an abortion. The baby's father didn't care one way or the other, and Sarah didn't have any idea what she wanted.

Over the course of several days, we discovered that Sarah wasn't even clear about how she had become pregnant, and we decided it was time for a customized version of Sex Education 101. Jackie had a good relationship with Sarah, so she decided to plunge right in.

Forty-five minutes later, Jackie emerged from Sarah's room,

looking like a truck had run over her and then backed up and ran over her again. She was annoyed. She was sad. She was discouraged. "She knows how she got pregnant all right. She knows all about the penis and vagina stuff. She just doesn't know *why* she got pregnant!"

"Why she got pregnant?" I asked. "She got pregnant because she had unprotected sex."

"Well, yeah, but there's more to it than that. Get this. Sarah went to her mom to talk about sex. Her mom told her ... I swear to god she says her mom said this ... her mom told her she wouldn't get pregnant if she had sex during a full moon. Guess what? She did, and she is!"

I couldn't believe it. Not that she got pregnant, but that people could pass along such information in the twenty-first century. "Her mother told her she wouldn't get pregnant if she had sex during a full moon? She must have been joking."

Jackie was already shaking her head. "I don't know if she was kidding or not; her mom's not too bright. But whether she was joking or she really believed it, the result's the same—Sarah's pregnant."

Most schools in the United States today have some form of sex education, ranging in quality from excellent to abysmal. Unfortunately, many teenagers see the classes as a blow off and prefer to believe what they learn from their friends, no matter how full of errors that information may be. In Sarah's case, she had received misinformation from her mother, whom she trusted, and no amount of sex education in the schools had been able to counter what her mother had told her.

When I was a teenager in the late '60s, becoming pregnant outside of marriage was not a good thing. It was neither a socially-acceptable, nor personally-desirable, choice. If by chance a pregnancy occurred, the young woman was faced with few choices.

Homes for unwed mothers generally provided safe pre- and post-natal care for the pregnant girl/woman and her child, as well as a safe and confidential home-away-from home. There was usually some sort of deception on the part of the young woman and her family—such as telling friends the young woman was visiting relatives out of state—in order to keep her pregnancy a secret, and this often led to feelings of shame on the part of the young woman. Typically, such homes allowed the mother to continue with her education and arranged for adoption of the infant immediately after birth. After her convalescence, the mother could pick up where she left off and continue on with her education and her life without the encumbrance of an infant.

Abortion was not an option in those years, at least not a legal one. For those pregnant young women with enough money, connections, and determination, abortions could be arranged in Puerto Rico or Mexico, and even in some large U.S. cities. Often performed under unsanitary conditions and without any type of anesthesia, most illegal abortions were both unsafe and degrading.

For women who wanted abortion but were unable to obtain one because of lack of money or opportunity, self-abortion became an option. Lye, soap, Lysol, and iodine douches, as well as self-inserted catheters, knitting needles, and goose quills, were common methods. These attempts were degrading and unsanitary, and sterility, or even death, was not uncommon. *Important note to readers: Do not try any of these methods to self-abort. You will die. Help can be obtained from Planned Parenthood at http://www.plannedparenthood.org/ (click on Find a Health Center).*

In some cases the young woman would deliver the baby and then turn the infant over to a relative to raise. Sometimes the maternal grandparents would even raise the child as a sibling to the biological mother.

The adolescent biological mother who kept and raised the infant herself was relatively rare, and keeping the baby usually meant the end of her education and a varying degree of dependency on her family for food, shelter, and childcare. A normal teenage social life and development were severely derailed.

Obviously, none of these options was ideal, but today's situation is no better. In fact, while the incidence of teenage pregnancy in the United States has actually declined in the last several years, our nation continues to have one of the highest teen pregnancy rates in the western world. And despite the prevalence of sex edu-

The Forgotten Future

cation programs in schools and the availability of reliable birth control, approximately three-quarters of a million teenage girls become pregnant each year. Our federal government spends the staggering sum of more than $40 billion dollars a year to provide social services to teenagers and their babies.

In our sexuality education groups, I frequently asked the kids, "Why do you think we talk to you guys about this stuff? Why do we care? Why the movies, the pamphlets, the opinions offered? I know you get it at school, too. Do you think we're just out to ruin your good time?"

Once they had recovered from my unintended double-entendre about "getting it" at school, their stock answer was usually *because you care about u*s. I think it was really intended to mollify me into believing they were all thinking maturely and acting responsibly about sex. I also believe it was designed to get me to stop talking about things that made them uncomfortable.

It didn't work. I knew that most of the kids that I worked with were awash in misinformation and misconceptions (no pun intended, I promise) about sexuality, and as I always told them, if you're old enough to do it, then you're old enough to talk about it. Or at least listen.

One of my most disheartening discoveries when discussing sex with the kids was to learn that for many young people sex is ... well ... just sex. It's an act. Something to do. The kids may or may not feel particularly fond of the person with whom they are so intimately involved, but across the board, there is no view of sex as an expression of profound love, of commitment, of passionate intimacy. Sexual intercourse is no longer seen as an expression of love reserved for one very special person. Rather, for many, it is little more than a handshake.

Accompanying this very blasé attitude about sex was another even more profound discovery: many teenage girls today actually hope to become pregnant while still in their teenage years and while still unmarried. They don't just think about it, fantasize about motherhood, dream about "someday ..." A significant number of teenage girls today either consciously, or unconsciously, plan to become pregnant.

STOP.

Deborah Clark Ebel, R.N.

Some girls "forget" to use any form of birth control, some say "It'll never happen to me", and some don't like the idea of planning for sex. They prefer to let romance sweep them away and just let "it" happen. Like in the romance novels. Then they're caught unawares and feel no responsibility when the "unexpected" arrives.

For those who deliberately become pregnant, reasons range from an attempt to show the world that they are grown up, to a desire to have someone love them, to bearing a child as a way to declare their independence and escape parental control.

Anytime I asked a group of teenage girls whether they had ever purposefully attempted to become pregnant, it was not unusual for a large number of them to say they had done so on at least one occasion. While this is by no means a scientific poll, it's alarming to discover how little understanding these girls have about the responsibilities of parenthood. It was also interesting to note that without exception these same young women told me that if TANF, AFDC, and other social services programs were not available, *they would never have considered becoming pregnant.*

It may be hard for adults to understand how these young women can be so misguided as to believe that they are in any way equipped for parenthood, but many fervently believe they are. They have no concept of the emotional or financial costs of parenthood, and while social service and other programs have helped many, perhaps it's time for us to consider whether these programs might actually encourage some to enter into parenthood prematurely to the detriment of mother and child and society. Perhaps another approach to the problem of teen pregnancy might be more effective.

*   *   *   *

Anyone meeting Elena and four-month-old Kyrie for the first time might presume the pair were a twelve-year-old baby-sitter and her charge. In fact, Elena was fifteen and engaged to seventeen-year-old Jeremy. Elena, Kyrie, Jeremy, and Jeremy's mother lived in a two-bedroom apartment close to the high school.

The Forgotten Future

Elena liked to show off her engagement ring and prattle on about her life with Jeremy. She enthralled the other girls with tales of being an independent adult. She carried around dog-eared copies of *Modern Bride* and *Brides* magazines and wistfully described the wedding she was going to have someday. At times, she adopted a somewhat superior, pseudo-grown-up, attitude toward her peers and on occasion even blatantly scorned what she called their "immature" behavior.

We never once heard her say she loved her baby.

She was exhausted and depressed. Jeremy was exhausted and depressed. We worried about Kyrie.

Each morning at home, Elena awoke at 5:00 to feed the baby before getting ready for school. At 7:45, Jeremy arrived home from his all-night job just in time to drive Elena to school and his mother to work.

He spent the morning and early afternoon taking care of the baby, and at 3:00 he left to pick up Elena at school. At 5:30, he had to pick up his mom from work—Elena wasn't yet old enough to drive. After a quick dinner, Jeremy would try to catch a few winks before leaving for his job at 10:30.

After she got home, Elena did her schoolwork and the laundry and helped Jeremy with the baby. Kyrie was one of those difficult babies who didn't sleep well, so Elena rarely got more than four hours' sleep before being awakened by the baby at 5:00 in the morning to begin the cycle again. As I said, she was exhausted.

She was caught in a situation that she hated and she didn't know what to do about it. She longed to be a teenager again, planning for the prom, going to parties, dreaming of the future. Her future, however, had already arrived—in a six-pound package.

*　　*　　*　　*

At dinner one evening, Abram sat next to Kelly and stroked her short hair. She giggled and said, "Don't!" in a voice and with a smile that invited, "C'mon. Do it again."

I confronted her. "Kelly, if you really don't want him to touch you, tell him directly. You're sending him mixed messages, and he's hearing what he wants to hear. Your words say 'no', but that's not the message that's getting through."

"Yeah, Kel. Just say no." Abram smirked. He somehow sensed she couldn't do it.

"Abram, *don't*." She broke into giggles, then tried to recover. "Don't keep touching my hair." She muffled her laugh with her hand.

"Don't touch me. I don't like it," I prompted.

"Don't touch me. I don't like it," Kelly echoed.

"Okay, I won't," acquiesced Abram, with a gentlemanly nod.

"It's hard," she whined.

"I never said it was easy."

Over the next week or so I worked with Kelly to help her become more assertive. She had trouble figuring out the difference between being assertive and being aggressive. Like a lot of girls, Kelly thought expressing her own wants and needs was somehow inappropriate and that she should subjugate her thoughts and opinions to please others. What I was discovering about her way of looking at things helped me to understand how the man at the railroad tracks was able to get her to pose for him so easily.

"Okay," I said. "Let's suppose you're in a parking garage or office building or some place waiting for an elevator. The elevator comes and the only person in the elevator is a guy. Maybe he looks a little creepy; maybe he looks okay. For whatever reason, you feel a little icky about getting on the elevator. What would you do?"

"I'd get in," she replied, as if there were no other option.

"Wrong! You stay right where you are. Don't get into a closed place in a situation you don't feel right about from the outset."

"But I wouldn't want him to feel bad or think I didn't like him."

"You don't know him, Kelly! You don't owe him anything. It doesn't make any difference whether he thinks you like him or not. Think about yourself." I was almost shouting, to equalize effect with content. "You can't put yourself at risk to avoid hurting someone's feelings. You could end up being a lot more than hurt."

She pursed her lips.

The Forgotten Future

"You're lucky that guy only took pictures. You know that?" It wasn't a question; it was a statement.

"I know, I know. Okay, but what could I say?" She looked genuinely perplexed.

"Well, you really don't have to say anything, but if you feel you absolutely, positively, must say something, then how about 'I'm waiting for someone' or even 'I'll wait for the next one'? There is nothing there to make anybody feel bad."

And to cover all her possible concerns, I added, "If someone does feel bad because you don't get on the elevator, that's his problem."

We role-played for a while. The closet was the elevator, and we took turns being elevator man and Kelly. We laughed. She said she could do it, but I still wondered.

*   *   *   *

Caitlyn sat under the dim night-lights at the end of the hall, ensuring that things stayed on the up-and-up. She had been at her post for at least half of her eight-hour shift, and I wanted to let her know that I would be off the unit for a short while and then would relieve her for a much-deserved break. "Everything's okay," she said as I approached. "The girls turned on their light after you told them not to and were talking, but they're quieter now."

I could hear soft whispering from room 410.

A noise from room 409 caught my attention, and I frowned as I tried to make out what was being said.

"Oh, he's just talking to himself. If he keeps it up I'll go in and tell him to quiet down," Caitlyn assured me. I stepped closer to the door and rested my ear against the crack between the door and the jamb. There seemed to be a conversation going on, but I could only catch an occasional word. *Taught. Why. God.*

I listened carefully. Was someone in there with Ricardo? As I held my ear to the door, I thought he might be praying. I felt like an intruder. Then I heard muffled crying and realized that he wasn't praying. He was talking to his best friend.

His closest friend since childhood had been killed a few weeks previously when he was hit by a car while crossing the street. Ricardo was there and saw it happen. He had seen the SUV coming, but had yelled too late to warn his friend.

I heard him cry out, "You taught me how to cross the street, to look both ways. Why didn't *you* look? If you had, you would still be here so we could look after each other. We were like brothers, man. Why? God, why? I wish it was me."

I glanced over my shoulder at Caitlyn and whispered, "I'm going in," and pulled open the door. The room was dark, and I couldn't see anything. It was quiet except for Ricardo's sobs.

"Ricardo," I called out, "it's Debbi. I'm going to turn on one of the lights."

No answer.

I reached for the switch and flipped up the first one.

Ricardo lay prone on the floor, head toward the door. His short black hair, damp with agitation, stuck straight out. Dressed in flowered boxers and a blue tee shirt, his arms were bent at the elbows and tucked tight to his sides. Toes pointed in. Except for his size, he looked like a little boy. I knelt near his head, wanting to reach out and calm him, to mother him and stroke his hair. Something kept me from doing so, either role or propriety, or what I knew of his past. I kept my hands at my side.

"Ricardo, were you talking to your friend?"

He nodded, almost imperceptibly.

"What was his name?"

"Angel."

"I'm sorry Angel died, Ricardo. I know it hurts." I paused, considering how much to share and what to say. Sometimes we share personal information and sometimes we don't. Sometimes it's a hard choice, and we have to make a quick call. For whatever reason, I decided to play it close and say very little. "I was exactly your age when someone I cared about very much died. I still think about him. Time helps."

His shoulders heaved, and he continued crying. More softly now.

I remained at his side and then gently reached out and touched his shoulder, ever so lightly.

The Forgotten Future

Ricardo didn't say anything for a long while, and we stayed in place on the floor. When you're seventeen and hurting beyond words, it seems like nothing will ever get any better. The concept of time as healer is incomprehensible.

Finally he spoke softly. "Can I be alone for a while?" He wasn't crying anymore.

I stood and looked down. "If you want to talk some more or anything, let me know, okay?" I still wanted to reach out and hold him close, as if he were my child, but I turned and walked to the door. "Light on or off?"

"I don't care."

The moon cast a bright glow through the window. I flipped the light switch down and opened the door. "G'night, Ricardo. Hang in there."

*   *   *   *

Abram had become more disruptive and inappropriate on the unit and in the drug education group. The drug and alcohol counselor grew frustrated as Abram failed to take any of the information about drugs seriously. While the heavy drug-using kids often thought the drug ed group was a joke, they usually at least gave lip service to the anti-drug message.

Not Abram. He liked his weed and let everyone know that he had no intention of giving it up. His only concession to what he considered our "tight-ass" attitude about drugs was surrendering his tee shirts emblazoned with pot leaves and images of drug paraphernalia. He sent them home with his dad and his stepmother when they came in for family therapy.

While reviewing the charts for doctors' orders one evening, I came across an order, the likes of which I had never before seen.

"Howard, have you seen this order that Dr. Carmichael wrote on Abram?" I turned around in the swivel chair and held out the chart to Howard. "You have to see this. I've never seen an order like this in my life."

He read the order and shook his head in disbelief. Handing the chart back to me, he said, "Never. I've been doing this for a lot of years, and I've never seen an order like that."

The order read:

Change pt chemical dependence tract to psychiatry tract.
Pt's father approves of pts recreational use of marijuana.
Do not make pt feel he's doing anything wrong.

(signed) Dr. Carmichael

Of all the drugs that are illegal in the United States, marijuana is the most controversial. While there are many people who support the legalization of small quantities for medical, personal, or recreational use, for the time being both the possession and use of marijuana remain illegal. My understanding of our role at Oak Haven, indeed the mission of Oak Haven itself, was to treat patients with mental health issues and promote behavioral changes to produce socially-acceptable and responsible behavior.

I wondered aloud, "What are we supposed to do? Just say 'Oh, okay, go ahead, Abram. Smoke pot. Use drugs. Whatever. No problem. You just go ahead and do whatever you want to do.'"

Alcohol and marijuana are what are called gateway drugs because they often lead to the use of stronger and more dangerous drugs. Whatever Abram's decision regarding the use of such substances might be after he became an adult, at thirteen he really wasn't mature enough to make such a choice.

Howard had it figured. "Carmichael's just afraid Abram's dad will pull him out of here if we make him too uncomfortable about the pot. If there has to be a choice between therapy and money, guess which wins?"

Carmichael had a lot of power at Oak Haven. Besides being the medical director, each year he admitted more adolescents to our unit than any of the other doctors. He had been known, when aggravated or aggrieved, to simply stop admitting patients to Oak Haven and admit his patients elsewhere. Money talks.

"I don't know what to say." I was speechless, which didn't happen often.

"I know what to say. Bullshit!" Howard was still shaking his head. "I've never seen anything like this. It's irresponsible."

I wondered how many other kids might try to pull the same sort of thing to get out of drug ed group or any other group or educational experience they didn't like or didn't want to face if they found out how easy it was to get over on the doctors.

I shook my head and returned to my charting.

*   *   *   *

Frankie was arguing with his state social worker when they arrived on the unit. His past twenty-four hours had been exciting, to say the least.

At sixteen, he was a long-term state custody kid, having been in more than a dozen foster homes and half that many treatment facilities. Two weeks previously, he had run away from his most recent foster home. He had spent the last couple of nights in a local shelter where he had raised hell, and the shelter director told Frankie that he had to leave. That didn't sit well with Frankie.

Sometime in the next few minutes, Frankie had slipped unnoticed into the shelter's infirmary and emerged carrying an empty bottle of lidocaine, a local anesthetic. He told the shelter director that he had swallowed the entire bottle.

The paramedics were called, and Frankie was rushed to the emergency room. Once he found out they were going to pump his stomach, his story changed to, "I didn't really swallow it, I just wanted attention", but it was too late. He got pumped anyway, and then he was released, unaccompanied. He took a cab back to the shelter, hoping the director would have a change of heart and allow him to stay. It didn't happen. He was told to leave immediately.

Frankie wasn't very happy, so he sneaked into an unoccupied office and did the first thing he could think of to get even: he called 911.

He told them he was being held hostage.

He gave them the address and hung up.

They believed him.

Frankie grabbed a wallet from a staff member's purse, escaped through the second story window, slipped to the ground over the porch roof, and ran away before the shelter staff even knew what had happened.

At this point I was frankly a little skeptical about the whole story, particularly the part about the 911 call, but the social worker assured me that it was all true. And I hadn't even heard the best part yet.

Taking Frankie's call at face value, the police hostage negotiation squad and SWAT team arrived at the shelter and surrounded it. The shelter director had absolutely no idea what was happening, or why, so it took a while to get things straightened out with the armed rescuers. After everyone had a better understanding of who the players were, things calmed down. The police picked Frankie up later in the day at a local game room, having been supplied with a photo taken when he arrived at the shelter. Child Protective Services was notified, and Frankie's social worker assisted with his transfer to Oak Haven.

Frankie thought it was a real hoot.

*   *   *   *

Crystale felt better after a few days in bed. Her bruises had turned a rather sickly yellow, and scabs had formed on the cuts around her nose and mouth. She wasn't quite as cranky anymore either, although I couldn't blame her after the way she had been beaten.

She was a cute girl who should have been going to junior high and hanging out at the mall with girlfriends. Flirting with pimply-faced boys wearing braces. But, instead, she really thought she had stumbled upon paradise, the stuff of dreams, when she found Benny.

Benny. The love of her life. The man of her dreams. Her knight in shining armor.

Her pimp.

Benny was twenty-six. They met at a party, and she liked him immediately. He treated her like a lady, bringing her drinks and joints all night long. Later they went back to his apartment where he made love to her slowly and lovingly and where, she says, he "made me feel like a woman". By the next morning, Crystale was in love and had agreed to move in with him.

They were together two weeks before he brought up being "short" for the rent and suggested that she could help him out by going to bed with a guy he knew. Although she was scared, she agreed, and then she did it again and again until she was turning tricks several times a day.

But at night, after the drunks and the dirty old men and the perverts, she would go home to Benny *because he loved her*. She knew that he loved her, she said, because he told her so.

Then she laughed because she realized how ridiculous that sounded and she went on to great lengths to explain that it wasn't just because he said it. He showed it.

"How? I asked."

"He says to me, "O-o-o-o baby, you so beautiful. You got the bestest body. You drive me wild. C'mere baby, I can't keep my hands off you. You are *perfect*!""

"Okay. Tell me more."

"He only hits me when I've done something wrong."

"Yeah, and ...?"

"He only sends me to johns he knows. He won't let me go with a stranger."

"Oh really? Well what about that old boozer you told me about, the one you said smelled like a wet dog?"

"Well, that was a special case, but usually Benny knows the guys and, besides, the money is good."

"But he takes it all."

"Not all of it. He gives me a place to live and clothes to wear, and he puts the rest in savings for me so I can buy a car when I turn sixteen."

Oh please ...

She wasn't the only young prostitute I worked with. Like Crystale, the others arrived at Oak Haven carrying beepers and cell phones and unpacking incredible lingerie, the likes of which I wouldn't have dared wear until I was long-married. I have even found sex toys in their bags. Unfortunately, there are far too many young women who have been wooed by a male convincing them to sell their bodies, while at the same time telling them how much he loves them. In order to prove their devotion to their man, they do whatever he wants. Such a life takes place in the seediest holes in town, with people you wouldn't invite into your living room.

She was only fourteen.

Chapter 7
Food for Thought

Anyone who has spent any amount of time around teenage boys knows that they like to eat. A lot. The hospital where I had previously worked provided three well-balanced meals every day and, in addition, kept a fully-stocked patient kitchen on the unit. There was decaffeinated coffee, tea and soda, assorted fruit juices, cheese, crackers, bread sticks, peanut butter and jelly, puddings, fresh fruit, Popsicles, dehydrated soups, and microwave popcorn available for snacks. Two evenings a week, the cafeteria staff sent up a special treat, such as trail mix, ice cream and toppings for sundaes, or vegetables and dip.

Oak Haven had a different philosophy. Although the meals served by the cafeteria were adequate, both in taste and portion, the patients' kitchen was kept barer than Old Mother Hubbard's. Every evening, the cafeteria staff sent up exactly enough small containers of juice and two packages of crackers for each patient for bedtime snack. The crackers were individually wrapped, bulk-purchase, and tasted like sun-dried cardboard.

With two sons of my own, I know most kids usually eat more than six dry crackers between supper and breakfast, and, at more than $1,000 a day, most parents could reasonably expect their child to have more than that, too. I don't mean shrimp cocktail or finger sandwiches, but a piece of fruit or some fresh bread and peanut butter and jelly would be nice.

The kids were hungry between meals. They complained, and I had to admit that they had a point. So, Jackie and I made it our personal mission to improve the unit snack situation. We actually thought it would be a fairly simple and straightforward task to requisition food to the unit kitchen for the kids. Nothing fancy, just basic stuff that kids like to eat.

We were wrong.

Our inquiries and requests were passed from person-to-person until, ultimately, we had spoken to half-a-dozen people, none of whom would give the go-ahead to improve the situation, and none of whom could explain their reluctance to give us what we wanted. Finally, they either got tired of hearing from us, or maybe we just contacted the right person, but we eventually found out why the kitchen didn't stock food on the unit for the kids.

"The staff will eat it," the clerk said simply.

"Excuse me?" I didn't think I had heard him correctly.

"If we leave food in the patients' kitchen, the staff will eat it or take it home and the patients won't get it anyway."

"You must be kidding." I could tell by the dour look on his face that he wasn't, but I had to pursue this. I couldn't believe what I was hearing. "You don't honestly think the nursing staff wants to do their grocery shopping in Oak Haven's patients' kitchen do you?"

He most certainly did. That explained why they always took such care to send up exactly the same number of cookies and juices as the number of patients. The unspoken message was, *"Don't you gluttonous, overfed staff think you're going to pig out on cookies at Oak Haven's expense. No siree, not gonna happen. We got your number. You got sixteen patients? Then you get sixteen cookies. Period."*

"No, I'm not kidding. We're not supposed to keep stuff up in the patients' kitchen because staff will use it up."

It took another week's haggling, but with input and assistance from the nutritionist as well as backup from several journal articles concerning the caloric and nutritional needs of adolescents, the cafeteria manager finally acquiesced and advised us that, henceforth, we would be permitted four loaves of bread per week and two jars each of peanut butter and strawberry jelly. Individual packets of saltine crackers would be available, as well as microwave popcorn, and, if the unit staff was willing to pick it up, we could even have fresh fruit three times a week.

The cupboards were still awfully bare for a unit full of teenagers, but it was a beginning. We staff, however, had to give our solemn promise not to touch so much as an apple.

*   *   *   *

The kids stared as Charlie exited the elevator. He might have been a rather nice-looking fifteen-year-old, but he suffered from some endocrine problems and, as a result, looked sort of, well … monkey-like.

He was small statured, and his closely-knit eyebrows formed something of a furry bridge across his face. A soft, dark down covered his cheeks. His voice was husky, and he always sounded like he needed to clear his throat. Even his doctor described him as looking like "some character out of Kubrick's *A Clockwork Orange*".

His parents had seen an Oak Haven promotion on the Internet and had brought him to the hospital hoping to get help with his increasingly aggressive, sometimes violent, behavior in the home. In addition to his angry outbursts toward both parents, he had threatened his brother with a meat cleaver. His parents didn't understand the dramatic changes in their formerly quiet, good-natured elder son and feared for the safety of their family.

Charlie was accompanied by his father and brother, and we sat together in one of the interview rooms doing admission paperwork. His dad struck me as extremely concerned about his son. Charlie, himself, was eager for admission because he realized things weren't going well at home and he wanted help "to change". He wanted to be normal and like other kids again.

I couldn't help but notice that Charlie's thirteen-year-old brother was already three or four inches taller and well on his way to becoming a handsome young man. His brother was pleasant and articulate and obviously very concerned about the changes in Charlie. The physical dissimilarities between the two boys were dramatic, and I wondered how much of Charlie's anger and aggression were fueled by the changes in his brother and the rapidly-widening gap between them.

The family understood the no-visitors/no-phone-calls-for-twenty-four-hours rule, but Dad promised Charlie that both he and Charlie's mom would be in to visit as soon as it was allowed. I assured him that we would take good care of Charlie and then allowed them a few minutes to say good-bye.

While they were talking, I shifted papers and wondered how the other kids were going to react to and treat Charlie. When Charlie and his dad and brother had stepped off the elevator, I saw a couple of kids nudge each other and barely cover their laughter behind their hands. Sometimes they could be caring and understanding of kids who were different, but at other times, and more frequently, they were cruel and hurtful. Knowing the group of kids we had as well as I did, I expected the latter. I sincerely hoped Charlie would be helped more than harmed.

*   *   *   *

Thirteen-year-old Carl thought about dying. Not just occasionally. Constantly. Obsessively. He planned his own death and the methods by which he would achieve it. He talked about it to anyone who would listen.

He idolized Kurt Cobain. Cobain of the musical group *Nirvana.* Cobain, who depressed and despondent, placed a shotgun to his head and pulled the trigger. Carl said he talked to Cobain and wished he could be with him. He said he didn't remember a time when he didn't think about dying.

When he was eight, he asked his sister to drown him in the family pool.

At nine, he tried to hang himself.

On his thirteenth birthday he took an overdose of sleeping pills.

And, just recently, he had gone into a public rest room at the mall and impulsively dyed his hair to match Cobain's. Now he was talking about getting a gun. A *shotgun.*

His parents were terrified.

*　*　*　*

"Yes ma'am, I did. Thank you very much."

I had just asked our new admission whether she had eaten dinner before coming to the hospital. She was so polite that I was taken aback. In a world where I was regularly called every abusive and degrading name that the imagination can conjure, it was a shock to be "ma'amed".

When I was fourteen, I moved from the southern United States to New England. Born and raised in the South by southern-born parents, "Yes ma'am" and "yes sir" rolled from my lips like butter off a hot biscuit. It was an automatic response and didn't require any forethought whatsoever. The way I had been raised, to omit the ma'am or sir was rude and carried with it the likelihood of reprimand from any adult within earshot.

So, when I visited a new "Yankee" friend one day and her mom asked if I would like something to drink, I quite naturally smiled and said, "Yes, ma'am, thank you". Well, you would have thought I had called her, well, something other than ma'am, because she became beyond angry. She stepped back and sarcastically replied, "Don't you 'yes ma'am' me, young lady. I don't have to put up with your smart-mouth crap!"

That was how I learned that those outside the South sometimes use "yes ma'am" in a mocking and rude way, sort of like "Oh sure, your royal highness". She assumed that that was what I was doing. Her daughter and I both tried to explain that politeness was part of my upbringing, but she would hear none of it. As far as my friend's mother was concerned, I was rude, and that was that. Her mother never liked me after that.

I hadn't met anyone as genuine and polite as sixteen-year-old Madison in a long time. She had a serious alcohol problem, drinking every day, just about all day. Heavy drinking. Hard-core drinking. She felt she had come to a crossroads and wanted to stop. Seriously.

Deborah Clark Ebel, R.N.

I accompanied her to an Alcoholics Anonymous meeting one evening, where she spoke eloquently of the pain and problems her drinking had caused her family and the embarrassing and dangerous situations into which she had placed herself when she was drunk. She wanted to get on with her life. She said she wanted to go to college and become a teacher. She wanted to grow and be and do.

Oh. There was one other little problem. She was pregnant.

*   *   *   *

William's psychosocial assessment revealed a long history of exhibitionism and sexual perpetration on younger children of both sexes. We had assigned him to a private room for other kids' safety and explained very clearly that such behavior would not be tolerated—and that included sleeping nude, which he insisted was the only way he could get to sleep.

William, sixteen, was reportedly sodomized at the age of eleven by a neighbor. While he denied ever having been molested prior to that time, that was hard to believe because his history of inappropriate sexual behavior with his siblings went back to his early childhood. It had to have started somewhere.

Some of the physicians' history notes pointed to William's continuing improper expressions of sexuality and included recommendations for extensive long-term therapy. Others saw William as simply misunderstood and suggested that he had been falsely accused. They considered it normal childhood exploration and downplayed its significance.

The family dynamics were fascinating. Extremely religious, William's parents encouraged their children to keep to themselves rather than make friends in their school and community. They didn't allow television in their home, nor did they allow the children to listen to commercial radio. When the children were in elementary school, the parents insisted that the children be excused from watching cartoons or fairy-tale videos, and when the children entered junior high, they did not attend family life classes. His parents preferred not to discuss sexuality with their children, but, when necessary, they euphemistically referred to anything sexual as "being unclean."

There had been extensive sexual play between William and his siblings, both younger and older. When he was in grammar school, he had been interviewed by a community psychologist after a teacher expressed concern about his behavior. William said he had "no idea" why children would want to look at, or touch, each other's "private parts". He asked several times, "When can we stop talking about this stuff?" and abruptly shifted the conversation to ask if he could shave off his pubic hair when it grew in.

The sexual play between brothers and sisters progressed to mutual masturbation, oral sex, and intercourse, and resulted in the siblings being placed in several different foster homes. William's sexual activity continued with children in the foster homes and in the neighborhood, and it was during this period of time that William was reportedly raped by a neighbor. At the same time, William's parents continued to deny any knowledge of their children's "unclean" activities.

Now that William was with us, though, I couldn't imagine what we could even begin to do to help him in such a short time. I did know, however, that I was going to watch him closely.

*   *   *   *

The quality of violence management training within psychiatric hospitals ranges from excellent to lamentable. Some hospitals design and conduct their own training classes, while others contract with local or national companies to provide training in the management of aggressive behavior. Staff members' responses to patients' threatening or aggressive behaviors greatly impacts the safety of the unit and everyone present.

It's important that training include techniques for dealing with a wide range of potentially dangerous and aggressive behavior, from abusive language to agitation to property damage or physical attacks on others or self. All of the techniques need to be understood and practiced regularly in order to deal with problems safely and effectively. Ideally, staff will have an understanding of the causes of limit-testing and acting-out, as well as cues or signals that a patient's behavior is escalating and that physical intervention may be required. Effective communication techniques and de-escalation methods should be stressed, as well as the appropriate use of physical and mechanical restraints such as the safety coat and wrist and ankle restraints. Safety of the patient should go hand-in-hand with the safety of staff.

New and inexperienced staff members at Oak Haven were often unprepared for working on the units, even after attending the required classes. Oak Haven's notion of violence management training consisted of a once-yearly lecture and a couple of hours spent discussing ways to recognize common signs of agitation and potentially violent behavior in our patients. Leather wrist and ankle restraints were passed around the group to practice locking and unlocking, and staff was cautioned sharply what not to do because it could "cause us (Oak Haven) to get sued". It was made abundantly clear that it was better for one of us to be injured than to cause a patient discomfort as the result of protecting ourselves. *I must stress here that different hospitals have different levels of quality of violence management training, and most hospitals with which I am familiar do a better job than that indicated above.*

Those of us who had worked in inpatient psychiatry for a while already had a pretty good idea of how to manage a violent situation with the safety of our patients as well as our co-workers and ourselves in mind. It wasn't always as simple, however, for the newcomers. While many hospitals have excellent violence management training programs, working in a violence-prone environment anywhere remains hazardous for staff and for patients, no matter the caliber of staff training.

*   *   *   *

Carl's psychiatrist, Dr. Trudel, was new to Oak Haven, and it showed. His charting was clear and to the point and gave a clear, succinct assessment of the patient's condition that included his rationale for continued inpatient placement. It was just the kind of documentation that made the state inspectors and boards of accreditation smile. More importantly, it gave the nursing staff information about how the patient was presenting to the doctor.

Dr. Trudel's notes on Carl read:

October 4 – Patient is quite dangerous and manipulative. Very theatrical at times. Speaks of poisoning self with carbon monoxide.

October 9 – Patient remains quite deadly if he were to be released from the hospital. Borderline personality tendencies underlie antisocial, depressive and aggressive behavior with sadistic traits.

October 14 – Increasingly depressed and moody, obviously still dealing with major life issues. Not safe outside of the hospital. No goals. No interests.

October 20 – Remains a danger outside the hospital. Learning the treatment system. No identity, no sense of purpose and no more than hedonistic impulses. Thematic Apperception Test is FULL of themes of murder and aggression suggestive of conduct disorder.

October 24 – Patient states "I don't think why die? I think why live? I can do whatever I want. Consequences are of no concern, as they won't matter. We'll all die eventually anyway."

Even more interesting, though disturbing, was the social worker's take on Carl's family therapy session. "This whole family is just incredibly dysfunctional," said Margie, delicately balancing her leather-bound Day Runner on one knee while trying to balance her coffee on the other. She turned a page, and the black liquid sloshed over onto her tailored wool slacks. She frowned at the spots and then chose to ignore them. "They're pretty well off. Dad's a lawyer with Morgan, Kelsey and Taylor, and Mom teaches a couple of classes over at the community college. Carl's one of two children. He has a seventeen-year-old sister, and his parents had one other child who died of SIDS before Carl was born."

I handed her a tissue. "So Mom and Dad must get really scared when he starts saying he's going to kill himself?"

"Thanks. Yeah." She put the coffee cup on the floor and dabbed at the spot on her pants with the tissue. "Yeah, well, anyway, he's been doing this since he was little. It's really weird. He has absolutely no emotional attachment to anybody in the family except his mom." She wadded the tissue and leaned back in her chair. "Have you read his psych report?"

She didn't wait for a reply. "It talks about how the whole family protects Carl from anything that might be disagreeable or stressful. Dr. Trudel used the phrase 'protects and insulates' to describe how the family indulges him."

Margie shook her head and sighed, then continued, "He's got a lot of power in the family. All he has to do is say he's going to kill himself, and everybody jumps in to make things nicey-nice for him."

"How sweet," I said.

"Interesting, though. Mom is really blaming dad for all of Carl's problems. Today, in the session, she was going off on dad because he spanked Carl when he was little. Not beat—spanked. On the bottom. She said Carl felt unloved and unwanted and it was all dad's fault."

"She said that in front of Carl?"

"Yes!. And Carl looked like he loved every minute of it." She took a couple of sips of the hot coffee and put it back down on the floor. "Dad feeds right into it, too. Said he has to take the blame for a lot of Carl's problems."

"Great. It always helps to know who to blame," I replied, facetiously. "How did Carl react to that? His dad taking responsibility for his behavior?"

"Actually, Dad had enough sense not to say that in front of Carl. He asked to speak with me privately, and we talked for a few minutes after Carl left to come back up to the unit. He seems to have a little insight, but he can't stand up to his wife or to Carl. That's the problem. He went on and on about how he and his wife have always tried to remove anything from Carl's life that might be unpleasant or that Carl wouldn't like. Things escalate higher and higher every time Carl doesn't like something."

Margie picked up her Styrofoam cup and stood to leave. "Carl can't take 'no' for an answer or stand any kind of frustration. When things don't go his way, he threatens to kill himself or makes an attempt. I told Dad we're afraid that one of these times he may actually kill himself unintentionally."

He was a very scary kid.

*   *   *   *

Ryan was a very angry kid. Considering his history, he had every reason to be.

He was fourteen, and with his extremely short-shorn hair and his propensity for wearing black—jeans, shirts and shoes—he projected hostility. He was a big kid, well over six feet and two hundred pounds. And muscular. He questioned every rule, every directive, every request. He didn't want to be in Oak Haven in the first place, and since I was assigned as his primary care nurse, he took an immediate dislike to me.

It seemed to be an authority thing with Ryan. He didn't like people telling him what to do. He didn't like people even making suggestions about what he should do. Ryan viewed every exchange with an adult, in any role, as a challenge to his autonomy. We weren't making any inroads because he refused to talk with anyone on the unit about anything.

The little we knew about Ryan came to us through history notes dictated by his doctor. Throughout his childhood, Ryan had been horribly abused, physically and sexually, by his biological father. The doctor's notes went into graphic detail about the abuse visited upon Ryan, and as I read them, I tried to imagine how any human being could do such things to another, let alone to a child. His own child.

Doctor's notes described the progression of Ryan's abuse. "Ryan states that when he was younger his father began using him for sexual purposes by putting his hand on his leg and gradually moving up until his father reached into Ryan's pants and began masturbating him. Before long, his father progressed to forcing Ryan to suck on his father's penis until his father ejaculated. Eventually, his father moved on to raping Ryan, which occurred regularly. Ryan further reports that on more than one occasion his father took off his pants and sat on Ryan's face, as Ryan says, 'rubbing his butt in my face'. Ryan reports his father would then fart and defecate in his face and get up laughing."

Incredibly, for a long time Ryan didn't realize his father's actions were abnormal, let alone bizarre. He had grown up with such behavior and had nothing to compare his home life to. He didn't know things like that didn't happen in every family.

When he eventually came to comprehend the extent of his father's brutality, his pain was intolerably deep. As a way of protecting himself from the pain of his childhood, he grew angrier and angrier at the world and didn't care who he hurt. Least of all himself. Indiscriminate sex and lots of heavy drugs were his daily fare, and his future seemed to hold more of the same.

This angry young man was the person who arrived at Oak Haven. Yet, while he pushed everyone away, including me, there was something there, a spark, a sort of inner strength that intrigued and challenged me. What I knew of his past was horrific, but, even so, I realized that we would never be able to fully understand what he had been through. He had somehow managed to survive but now seemed to be at a point where he would have to make a choice: either clean up his act and make some dramatic changes or continue on the way he was going and end up in jail. Or worse.

*   *   *   *

Robin began report with our new patient. "April is thirteen, and she's in room 410A. She's Dr. Trudel's patient, in with diagnoses of dysthymia, alcohol abuse, and parent/child problem. Her mom brought her in, um … I guess a family friend recommended Oak Haven after April was suspended for drinking beer on school property."

I nodded and made a few notes on my report sheet.

The Forgotten Future

"She's been increasingly defiant and oppositional at home, and two days ago she got into a big physical fight with her mom. April says her mom beat her with a broom during the fight." Robin turned her left elbow and pointed to an area on her arm. "She has some bruising and swelling on the elbow where she says her mom hit her."

So far it sounded like stories I had heard more times than I could count: a kid acts out, the parent gets ticked off, and they come to blows. A parent hitting a child with a broomstick is never right, but I understood how at wits' end the parents sometimes felt when they no longer had control over their child's behavior. Many parents need to learn more appropriate ways of disciplining their children, but it's especially difficult when those parents were themselves abused as children.

"Now, this is where things get really complicated." Robin leaned forward. "Dr. Trudel says Mom is really pissed at April. He says she alternates between distancing herself and going ballistic at April *ever since April shot and killed her ten-year-old brother about a year ago.*"

"Ummm," I murmured, shaking my head from side to side and listening carefully. "That would complicate things. How'd it happen?"

"Well, April says that it was an accident, but I guess they're not so sure. There were four kids in the family, and April says she always felt left out, like she wasn't really a part of the family. This one afternoon her mom left April and her brother, Kyle, home alone and told April to clean the house. April was mad, and she locked Kyle outside. He kept trying to come in, screaming and crying and pounding on the door, so she took a gun out of a closet, worked the bolt action, aimed the gun at Kyle, and pulled the trigger. He was hit in the head and killed instantly. She says she only wanted to scare him."

My stomach turned, and I looked up and around at my coworkers, trying to gauge their reactions. Howard had stopped writing and sat expressionless, chewing on the end of his pen. Jackie's elbow was on the desk, supporting her head in her hand, eyes closed. I wondered how hearing of tragedies like April's had become so commonplace to all of us that they were almost routine. Such stories no longer jolted or surprised, and I was dismayed to know that I had become so inured to tragedy that things like this no longer carried any kind of shock value. I reflected for the umpteenth time on how society as a whole seemed to be so unaware of the crisis in our midst, and I was saddened that I had no answers, that no one seemed to have any answers.

*   *   *   *

Madison sat with her feet on the chair, hugging her knees and rocking back and forth. Her face was red, and an occasional tear ran down her cheek. I caught snippets of conversation, such, "What do you want me to do?" and "Why not?" and "What about Dad?" She was on the phone with her stepmother, Helen, and while it was obvious the conversation was unpleasant for her, the actual content remained a mystery.

Madison was approximately nine weeks pregnant, and when we had talked the night before, she disclosed that the father of her baby was Helen's fourteen-year-old son. He visited every other weekend and appeared to fit in well in this blended family. Helen didn't yet know the extent of her son's involvement with Madison; all she knew was that Madison was pregnant. Obviously she would have to be told the truth soon, and I suspected that the news would be devastating for everyone.

Suddenly, Madison hung up the phone and burst into tears, covering her face with her hands. Jackie walked over and gently rubbed her shoulders and smoothed her hair.

After a time Madison looked up at Jackie and drew in a deep breath. "Can we talk for a few minutes? Down in my room?"

Jackie nodded and held out her arm to Madison who slipped into the hug and buried her head under Jackie's chin. They turned and walked slowly toward room 406.

*   *   *   *

Charlie's parents visited regularly. A week or so after he was admitted, his father asked to speak to me. He said that he had noticed that a lot of the other kids never had any visitors. I had to admit that was true and told him that Charlie was fortunate to have parents who cared about him and showed it. All kids, even the toughest and most hardened, need to know that someone, somewhere, cares about them. We talked for quite a while, and it became clear that Charlie's parents were painfully beginning to understand and acknowledge that their elder son might never live up to their vision for his future.

The hopes that almost every parent has for his child.

The dreams parents dare to dream for their children.

The hopes and dreams that most likely would never come to be, at least not for Charlie.

But they loved him unconditionally.

Charlie's dad remarked that the next night was their younger son's birthday and asked if it would be all right if the family brought in an ice cream cake to share with the other kids on the unit. I was delighted to learn that they wanted to involve the entire unit and assured him that the kids would love it.

On Friday evening, the family brought in an old Jim Carrey comedy for the unit, the birthday cake, and a huge box of microwave popcorn. The kids were excited, although I overheard a couple of disparaging comments about the movie being "stupid" and "boring". We only allowed movies rated "G" and "PG", but most of the kids had been viewing "R", and in some cases, "X" movies outside the hospital for years. There were a few comments about watching a "baby" movie, but, for the most part, the kids were polite and kept it together. Three or four of the kids went out of their way to thank Charlie's mom, and I heard a couple of them say they wished that their parents cared enough to do something similar.

When I returned on Monday following my weekend off, I learned that the weekend nurse had expressed concern about Charlie's parents trying to "buy" Charlie's acceptance into the group. She contacted Charlie's doctor, who in turn called Charlie's parents and asked them not to visit so often and especially not to bring in things for the other kids.

I felt bad for Charlie and his parents. Maybe they were trying to ease the way for Charlie, maybe not. My impression was that they were two caring and concerned adults who genuinely wanted to reach out to kids about whom not many others cared.

But we existed in a world of dysfunction, where every behavior was pathologized and where there was a veiled reason for everything. There was no room for genuineness, no room for sincerity. No room for giving without expecting something in return.

After that, the family visited, but kept to themselves. It seemed to me that everybody lost, but most especially, the kids.

*   *   *   *

Madison had more courage than I had seen in a long time. She also had an abundance of common sense, something sorely lacking in many of the situations with which we worked.

Her pregnancy had her caught between the proverbial rock and a hard place. Her stepmother had learned that her son was the baby's father and adamantly refused to allow Madison to return home to carry the baby to term. She was convinced that to allow Madison to have the baby—even if she adopted out—would cause problems for her son and ruin his future. She droned on about how her son had plans for college and shouldn't be, couldn't be, burdened with a child who would be out there "somewhere", how she wasn't ready to be a grandmother, and that Madison should have kept her legs together. Madison's father supported whatever his wife wanted.

We talked. Madison cried. She knew she couldn't possibly bear the child without some sort of family support and felt she was being pushed into having an abortion that she didn't want. Her stepmother and her father repeatedly told her that she was bad and thinking only of herself. I was sorry her parents didn't realize what an exceptional young woman they had in Madison, and I was annoyed that they, or anyone, would condemn her for her pregnancy. As I told Madison, she had done nothing more than millions of other girls do every day, only she had gotten caught. She was pregnant.

We spent a lot of time talking. I watched her cry. I told her she shouldn't ever let anyone tell her she was a bad person. We discussed how many young girls become pregnant on purpose in an attempt to prove their maturity or to have someone to love without considering the practical aspects of raising a child, thinking only of what they wanted at that moment.

She was a teen who was about as far from thinking only of herself as I had ever seen. Still, she was running out of options, running out of time. During one of our later talks I made a discovery that really aggravated me.

I had been wondering about the family makeup, about such things as how long the stepmother had been around, how long they had been married, how well did they usually get along, was she usually supportive—all things to try to get a feel for how things were at home. Then Madison told me that her father and "stepmother" weren't married after all, but had only been talking about it.

Well, that's okay, lots of couples these days aren't married and that's not for me to judge, anyway. I've seen some of those unofficial parents encourage and nurture far better than biological ones. But when I found out that Madison's father had only known the "stepmother" for four months, yet was willing to put his only daughter out of the house in deference to his "wife", I was stunned.

I had come to know a sensitive and sensible young woman who wanted to hurt no one, who only wanted to do what was right. She realized that she was still very young and couldn't raise a child alone. She knew she couldn't even carry the baby to term in order to adopt out without family support. She didn't want to abort. She believed abortion was murder.

But as options closed off to her and she had to come face-to-face with the harsh realities of her situation, she finally and tearfully simply said, "I guess I'll have to go along with what they want. I'll have to get an abortion." And that was that.

*   *   *   *

We had a new admission coming, and from the crisis worker's report he was going to be a handful. He had a long history of psychiatric and judicial involvement that made Oak Haven seem like Disneyland. From Ashley's description, I just about expected Ivan the Terrible. Instead, Ashley showed up with a neatly-dressed, handsome fourteen-year-old named Nick.

Nick was pleasant and polite as we began the admission interview. He had obviously been through a lot of them before. He knew all the terminology and had all the right answers. He knew the right things to say and how to say them.

I liked him instantly.

My internal warning signals immediately went into overdrive. I was used to working with kids who were oh-so-charming and very adept at pretense and manipulation, especially with adults, and I knew he must have had a lot of practice. And when they are so charming, even professionals have to be very careful to guard against being taken in.

We got to the part of the interview where I asked about previous hospitalizations and placements. He had been at Longmeadow, Western Hills Hospital, a couple of state facilities—including juvenile detention—and a few foster homes. He hadn't been at home for more than a month at a time since he was eight years old.

"Home" was his dad's four-room apartment. After Nick's mom died when he was seven, his dad was left to manage Nick and then thirteen-year-old Nadine. Their dad was a compulsive gambler who made frequent out-of-state trips to the popular gaming spots, leaving Nick at home in Nadine's care. Nick was still a little boy who missed his mother and very much needed his father. He began acting-out at school and became more than young Nadine could handle at home alone.

Fed up, Nick's dad called Child Protective Services, declared Nick uncontrollable and said he couldn't cope with the responsibility anymore. Eight-year-old Nick was placed into his first foster home.

I sat in the desk chair as Nick sat on the end of the bed and continued a lengthy, yet fairly succinct, narrative of his various placements, concluding with his arrival at Oak Haven. Then he smiled and shrugged his shoulders. "Now I'm yours," he said.

The Forgotten Future

*   *   *   *

Stefanie and Koryn had both been with us before. Several times. As a matter of fact, separately, they had each spent much of the past year with us, off and on. They were sisters, thirteen and fifteen respectively, but this was the first time they had been admitted together. This time we were holding them until we could find a permanent residential placement for them. They didn't know that, though. They assumed that they would be discharged back home in a few days and they could promptly run away again. Both girls hated any kind of authority and asserted that they should be able to live their lives any way they wanted.

Koryn, the elder of the two, had been the first to run away. The first time was when she was twelve and she and her parents had argued over something long-since forgotten. Early on, her parents would call the police and seek their assistance in finding her and bringing her back home. After the authorities brought Koryn back home, there would again be arguments with her parents, she would threaten them, they would ground her, and she would run away. This cycle had been pretty continuous since then.

At thirteen, Koryn continued running away, despite her parents' attempts to seek help from a therapist and from their minister. Her parents enrolled her in after-school activities, as well as her church youth group, but none of it made any difference. Koryn wasn't interested in such things.

At fourteen, she casually mentioned to a teacher at school that her parents were abusing her. No specifics, no details. Just "abusing". The teacher was required by law to report such an allegation to her superiors, which she did.

The school reported it to Child Protective Services, who investigated the family thoroughly. Neighbors were interviewed. Relatives. School officials. Church officials. Younger sister, Stefanie, and younger brother, Todd. After Child Protective Services determined that there was no validity to Koryn's charges, the file was closed.

Her mother became depressed, and her parents argued over

how to handle the situation. Koryn continued to run away and started to hang out with older kids. Drug users and other types. When she was fourteen and Stefanie was twelve, Stefanie ran away for the first time with her sister. Both girls disappeared for weeks at a time. Soon Stefanie joined her sister in making allegations of abuse against their parents.

The Child Protective Services investigatory process began again with a vengeance. Teachers. Clergy. Neighbors. Pediatrician. Friends. Family. Both parents were distraught. Same conclusion. File closed.

The girls continued to run away. Their father heard a rumor that Stefanie was staying in a crack house, so he went there himself, alone, to bring her home. He found Stefanie, but he also found her friends. He was beaten to a bloody pulp and left unconscious as Stefanie and her friends fled.

Feeling they had no choice but to place the girls in a safe place, i.e., a residential treatment facility, the parents and several adult friends found the girls and brought them to Oak Haven for their own protection until arrangements could be made to send them out of state. Both girls were placed on unit restriction and confined to wearing hospital pajamas and slippers. All clothing, including shoes, were confiscated and locked away in storage, lest the girls try to slip off the unit and back to the streets.

*   *   *   *

The last admission of the evening was on his way up. He was fifteen, and six months previously he had shot himself in the head with an air-powered pellet gun. The little information we had indicated he had been a popular and extremely bright young man before his suicide attempt left him functioning permanently at a preschool level.

His parents were having trouble handling his angry outbursts at home and needed assistance in coping with the changes in their son. He frequently flew into rages and trashed whatever was close by. At school he was becoming more and more troublesome and had difficulty following directions. Some of his teachers were intimidated; some were frankly frightened. In addition to all this, he was clinging and touching others in sexually-inappropriate ways. The way a preschooler might, without inhibition or constraint, but with the stature and appearance of a young man.

We were to keep him for a couple of weeks and try to change some of his more overtly inappropriate behaviors. Then we would send him off to a rehab facility in one of the southern states where, we were told, they were doing some groundbreaking work with head injuries.

The whole thing was tragic, and I wondered what had driven him to shoot himself. Then, I heard a rustling and looked up to see a pair of beautiful brown eyes and the broadest grin I've ever seen. He reached across the counter to shake my hand. "Hi! I'm Timothy. Who are you?"

Chapter 8
The Beat Goes On

T he full moon. Scientists tell us it's just one of the phases of the moon. They'll even go so far as to assert that it regulates the tides. But suggest that it influences the actions and behaviors of people, and they'll scoff.

On the other hand, ask any emergency room doctor, obstetric nurse, or mental health worker, and you'll get an earful.

Whether based in fact or folklore, happenstance or circumstance, there seems to be an abundance of unpredictable and acting-out behaviors during this particular lunar phase. Tempers flare, hormones rage, aggression and irrationality are the rule. It's a time to be extra vigilant.

From the admission report that accompanied Tyrone, it looked like he might be with us for a while. He had been in numerous fights over the past several months, and earlier on the day of his admission, his mother had found a loaded .38 under his mattress. His explanation was that he needed the gun to protect himself because some kids had threatened to beat him up. His mother didn't believe him and neither did I. He didn't strike me as scared; he seemed angry at the world.

His mom brought him in and stayed during our initial interview, and it was then that I learned that she had told him she was bringing him to Oak Haven to talk to someone about his temper.

She had promised him he wouldn't have to stay, that he was coming here just to talk to someone.

She lied.

Now, that's always a double-edged sword. My personal preference is that the kids be told where they're going and why. On the other hand, there are lots of kids who would just disappear if given warning. It's probably six of one kind and half a dozen of another. If a teenager really needs psychiatric help, he needs to get it, and I guess a little deception is acceptable in order to get him to a place where he can receive it. And if an adolescent needs to be placed within the juvenile justice system, parents need to be willing and able to call upon the proper authorities to pick him up.

It's a tough call, and parents usually don't feel very good about any of it. Kids threaten to never speak to their parents again or tell them they will hate them forever. Lots of guilt and lots of manipulation. Parents may feel that they have let their kids, and themselves, down, but I have always told the parents that I have worked with that if their child is in trouble and needs help, not to let their child's anger hold them back. Many years ago, I heard someone say that sometimes you have to love your kids enough to let them hate you. Or at least get mad as hell. I always thought that was good advice.

In any event, Tyrone and his mother were sitting with me in our interview room and he was very unhappy. Dressed in baggy clothes and backward baseball cap, he was neat and clean. He spoke little, but chose instead to communicate with me via nasty looks and the use of select four-letter words.

After a great deal of wheedling and coaxing by his mom, as well as subtle persuasion on my own part, he agreed to stay for the night. But first, he insisted, he had to call his girlfriend. Mom nodded and said, "The woman in the admitting office said it would be okay."

Uh, oh.

Oak Haven didn't have an "admitting office" as such. She was talking about the crisis worker who knew our rules about phone calls. All too frequently, the crisis workers and the physicians made promises to the kids and their parents that they knew would never be kept. The patient would then come up to the unit expecting to be able to do certain things, and then one of the nurses or MHTs would have to deliver the bad news that we couldn't permit. whatever it was that they had been told they could do.

Making phone calls was a big issue. The rule at Oak Haven was that no phone calls were allowed at all—not to anyone, not even parents—for the first twenty-four hours. After that, phone calls to parents were okay, but it would be a while before calls to friends—including boyfriends and girlfriends—were permitted. I knew it was sometimes tough on the kids, but that was the rule, and to make even one exception to a rule set us up for problems with every other patient on the unit.

So with this in mind that I, as tactfully as possible, let Tyrone know that he could not call his girlfriend. I even suggested that his mom call her to deliver a message or perhaps he could write his girlfriend a letter.

"Fuck this shit, man. I ain't staying here!" He stood and bolted around the table before I realized what was happening. He passed behind me, shoving my upper body slightly on his way to the door.

I jumped up and ran after him, yelling loudly, "Howard! Howard! I need help!"

Howard rushed into the hall from one of the patients' rooms and watched as I followed Tyrone through the double doors to the elevators. Tyrone pushed the elevator call button, and I stepped between him and the door.

"Tyrone, come on. Let's go back in and talk about this. Come on. This isn't going to work. Look, let's just go back in the interview room, and I'll explain why we have the rule. It'll just be a few days 'til you can call her." I stood back against the elevator door and assumed my most non-threatening stance while giving him some space.

The elevator hadn't arrived yet, but I heard the gears clanking and clanging and knew I had only a few seconds. I looked past Tyrone and saw Howard come through the double doors and stop. Waiting. Watching. Giving me a chance to try to convince Tyrone to return to the unit.

Tyrone paced back and forth, breathing hard and fast. Shaking his head, clinching his fists, he muttered something, but I couldn't make out what it was. I continued speaking softly, trying to de-escalate him.

The little "ding" signaled the elevator's arrival as it settled into place. The doors slid open.

"Tyrone ..."

He moved toward me. I stepped backward into the elevator, re-flexively holding my arms out in front, but he continued coming at me. Before I realized he wasn't going to stop, Tyrone had shoved me hard into the side of the elevator and I sagged to the floor. I saw the proverbial stars, but through the haze, I saw Tyrone push the elevator button.

Everything moved quickly after that, with lots of shouting and activity. Howard rushed into the elevator and pushed Tyrone to the back. "I've got him! It's okay, I've got him!" They struggled in the corner, amid grunts and groans.

It took me a minute to realize what had happened. I was dizzy and things seemed a little out of focus. When I pulled myself up off the floor, I shouted out, "Call Dr. Strong!" Caitlyn was already on the overhead as the elevator door closed, and I heard, "Dr. Strong to the elevators! Dr. Strong to the elevators!" echoing through the halls. The elevator started moving.

Still unsteady, I moved to help Howard. He and Tyrone strug-gled in the tight space, and Howard warned me, "Stay back, dam-mit! I've got him."

The elevator came to an abrupt halt on the third floor. The doors opened, and our Dr. Strong response was there, waiting to board. The same thing happened on the second and first floors. By then, the elevator was full, but Tyrone was still struggling. I pushed the button for the fourth floor, and the elevator started moving again.

Once back on the fourth floor, Tyrone seemed to have gotten his second wind, because he started fighting hard again, despite having six men working hard to subdue him. I climbed over the mound of grunting, sweating beings, grabbed one of the MHTs, and we went to the seclusion area to ready a bed for restraints. We wheeled the bed back to the elevator where we found five men and Tyrone on the floor, half-in, half-out of the elevator. They were lying still now, in a large heap.

They were so entangled that no one knew precisely how to begin to move Tyrone into restraints. He was somehow able to free one of his legs, and I caught a glimpse of his foot going straight into Howard's abdomen. Howard winced in pain, and the entire human mountain shifted. With that momentum, the men were able to lift Tyrone, kicking and swearing, spitting and threatening, onto the bed. It seemed to take forever to get the restraints in place and locked before Tyrone was finally moved to the seclusion area.

After the fracas had calmed, I went to console Tyrone's mother who was in a near panic at seeing her son assaulting people and being restrained. She cried for a good while and kept repeating, "I can't believe he did that! He's really a good boy. I can't believe it ..."

After she left, it was time for me to get the necessary doctor's orders, do the requisite paperwork for the restraint and seclusion, and return to the regular business of the unit—caring for the kids.

And time to convince Howard to go home, with a strong suggestion he stop in at the emergency room, since he could hardly walk.

And time to discover that Randall had also been hurt in the scuffle.

And time to file incident reports for their injuries.

And time to get someone in to cover the remainder of the shift for Howard.

I barely had time to notice that I had a pounding headache.

Before Howard left for the evening, though, I asked him why he did the takedown the way he did. Only then did I learn that after Tyrone shoved me into the wall, he had pulled back his fist to slug me full force in the face. Having had the wind knocked out of me, I had no idea what was happening, but Howard saw that I was about to be attacked and took Tyrone down. In his mind, there was no choice to be made. His attitude was simply, "None of my nurses is going to get hurt if I can help it."

Howard called later that night to tell us that he had stopped in at the emergency room. "I was driving home and it hurt so damn much I figured I better go." He had a way of phrasing things so that he was actually shrugging off any troubles. I knew he must really have had significant pain to actually go see a doctor. He sounded apologetic when he told me that he had two cracked ribs and would be out for a few days. I assured him that we would miss him, but things would be fine and he should stay home and recover.

When I thought about the evening later, I was very sorry Howard had been injured but I was profoundly grateful that he had been there for me.

*   *   *   *

Monday. 3:05 p.m. "You guys are gonna have a busy night," Robin warned at report. "It's been nuts here all day. The kids are totally off the wall. No one wants to do any work. It's just crazy." She threw up her hands in exasperation.

Caitlyn nodded her understanding, and I knew each of us was pondering what the evening might bring. While listening to Robin, I glanced up from my notes and through the window in the door I saw Tyrone entering the community room. Considering the ruckus he had caused the night before, I was a little surprised to see him having free rein of the unit. We'd have to keep a close eye on him.

Robin continued. "George is in room 404A, Dr. Evans' patient in with diagnoses of bipolar and polysubstance abuse." She looked up from her notes. "Dr. Evans has ordered that George's Uncle Martin cannot come in to visit him anymore."

"Oh, really? How come?" George's Uncle Martin was the only real family George had. He visited two or three times a week and had taken George out on pass a couple of times.

"You're not gonna believe this." Robin rolled her eyes. "Uncle Martin felt sorry for George and brought him in some weed. George says he only smoked half a joint, and he turned the rest in to Margie. Who knows? Anyway, Uncle Martin is *persona non grata* around here."

Report continued, and we moved on to Timothy. "Timothy," sighed Robin. I don't know what we're going to do about him. He

~ 174 ~

keeps touching the other kids inappropriately and I really thought Tyrone was going to punch him today."

"And then he says, 'I'm sorry', right?"

"Yes! He keeps saying, 'I'm sorry' every time he's redirected. It's constant. But then he turns around and does it again. Absolutely no short-term memory." She thought for a second. "He put his hand on Tyrone's thigh today and started rubbing it. He's gotta stop doing stuff like that or somebody is really going to let him have it."

Randall from maintenance knocked lightly on the door, then opened it and peeked in. "Can I interrupt for just a minute?" He glanced around, and his eyes finally settled on Robin. "I finished nailing the window in room 407 shut. Do you want me to do anything else while I'm here?"

Robin shook her head.

With no idea what was going on, Howard and I exchanged glances. We'd wait. Robin would get to it.

She caught our looks and said, "Victor has been throwing things out of his window all day. Papers, linen, books. Anything and everything. Dr. Carmichael said to nail it shut."

"Isn't that some kind of fire-code vio …?"

Howard's foot nudged mine. His eyes said *forget it*.

"Yeah. Probably. Carmichael's the medical director though, and if he wants it nailed, it gets nailed." She picked up her papers and resumed report.

I listened with one ear, still musing over the nailed window. The windows only opened a few inches anyway, to prevent anyone from jumping. Nailing the window no more trapped people inside than if it were not nailed. There was something that just didn't feel right about having the window nailed, though. Robin was right about one thing: if Carmichael wanted it nailed, it was nailed.

We finished report and walked toward the door. Robin stopped and turned to face me. "I guess you probably haven't heard yet, but we found out today that Timothy wrote a suicide note just before he shot himself."

"Oh yeah? Did he say why he did it?"

"Because he didn't want to hear his parents fight anymore; he said their arguing and fighting was tearing him apart, and it hurt too much. He thought the only way things would change would be if he died."

I wondered if they still fought ...

*   *   *   *

Tuesday. 3:10 p.m. Robin said in report that it had been another bad day and told us to prepare for a tough evening. Lately, we had been hearing that more and more frequently. She gave a brief discourse about our current kids being more delinquent than psych and ended with the news that the tape recorder that we used to tape report for the night shift had been stolen. The number one suspect was Elisabeth, who had been discharged earlier in the day.

Robin then told me that Becca's mother was waiting at the front desk to take Becca home. Becca was a fifteen-year-old who had taken a serious overdose after breaking up with her boyfriend. The combination of Pyridium, Robaxin, aspirin, Amitriptylin, Flexeril, and Indocin stunned even those of us who had experience with countless suicide attempts.

She was unresponsive when the rescue squad arrived, and the emergency room report indicated she was comatose when she got to the hospital. Emergency Room notes indicated her pupils were 2-4 mm and fixed, reactive to light but not accommodation. She had no gag reflex, no spontaneous movement, minimal deep tendon reflexes, her toes were pointed down. Her pulse was 130, blood pressure 105/51, respirations 24 and shallow, rectal temp 96.2. Glasgow Coma Scale score was IV.

In other words, she was in pretty serious shape. Miraculously, after a few days in intensive care, including two days hooked to a ventilator, she was medically cleared. Becca was transferred to Oak Haven, where she spent less than forty-eight hours. She abruptly decided that things were really much better in her life now and she would like to go home, thank you very much.

Dr. Trudel refused to discharge her because he didn't think she was ready to go home, so it would have to be an AMA discharge—against medical advice. This meant that while she was not seen to be an imminent danger to herself, in her doctor's opinion she needed treatment and his advice was that she should remain in the hospital.

The staff consensus was that considering the seriousness of her attempt as well as a recent abortion and her parents' divorce, the risks involved in discharge were too high. Trudel was the doctor, however, and his decision to allow her to leave AMA stood. Robin said she would take care of the discharge, including paperwork and notification of the administration about the AMA, before she left for the evening.

We finished report, and Robin stood up. "Oh, I almost forgot. Ryan's back in the seclusion room, clamoring to get out. He's getting agitated again, but I told him he'd have to wait until you could talk to him and process him out."

"Yeah. Right. Just as soon as I can get to him. Who's the rest of the staff?" I asked. So far, there were only Caitlyn and Barry and me. It was almost half-past the hour and even allowing for traffic, Jackie or Howard should have arrived by now.

Robin looked away and bit her lower lip. "You don't have any more staff for tonight. Howard's still out with injuries and they floated Jackie to the adult unit." She shrugged and added, "Sorry".

I'm sure my face betrayed my feelings, if not my thoughts, because Robin held up her hand and quickly added, "I know, I know. We tried to get someone, but no one's available."

"It's not your fault, Robin. I know that. It's just that with fifteen kids and the way things have been around here lately … I'm supposed to do an anger group tonight, but I'm not going to be able to do it. There's not even enough time to get to talk to all the kids, forget about doing anything therapeutic. It's not right. It's not safe." I shook my head and sighed. "You know, sometimes I feel like we're doing little more than babysitting." I wasn't telling her anything she didn't already know.

Tuesday. 3:45 p.m. We moved toward the door, and Robin turned. "Nicole has a 4:30 appointment at the medical center for an X-ray. She's been complaining that her right hand hurts, and Dr. Evans said to send her over and have it checked. There's a cab coming to pick her up, and an MHT from the adult unit will escort her over and back."

Nicole was a former patient who had been readmitted that morning. I had noticed her in the hall when I arrived to start the shift. She had a bad habit of smashing her fist into walls whenever she was angry, and that was probably the cause of her pain.

Report over, I headed toward the nurse's office and saw Nicole sitting on a chair just outside the office door. Purse in her lap, twisting her hair around her finger, she clutched a white toy rabbit. She was wearing her coat and was ready to go.

"Hey! How ya doing?" I greeted her.

She managed a weak smile and mumbled, "Okay, I guess."

I paused at her side and said, "Not so good, huh? Maybe we can talk when you get back from X-ray?"

Nicole nodded, and I smiled and moved on. It was getting late, and I knew I had at least two 4:00 meds to give—a Ritalin and an insulin—so I grabbed the med book and started checking orders. I looked over at the seclusion room monitor screen and saw Ryan mouthing obscenities and giving the finger to the camera.

"I told him you'd be in to talk to him after report," Robin reminded me, motioning toward the monitor.

"He'll have to wait unless you can get in there before you leave," I sighed. "I have to do meds first, and I can only do what I can do." I glanced up as Sylvia, the children's unit day nurse, pulled up the extra chair and sat down.

"Terrence's mom may come in and try to take him out of here tonight. She called today, making a lot of threats because we had reported her to Child Protective Services."

"Okay," I nodded. "You do know that it's only me and Caitlyn and Barry here tonight?" I asked.

"Yeah." Sylvia shook her head in that same, resigned, what-can-we-do look that had become all too familiar and continued. "We heard Terrence's mom was in the parking lot earlier today and had a shotgun in the back seat of her car. The receptionist downstairs has a description of her, and if she shows up, they're calling Child Protective Services and the police. Hopefully, she'll never get up here."

"Hopefully," I repeated, shutting the med book. I went into the med room and started unlocking the narcotics cabinet. I leaned back out the door and called to Sylvia, "Who's the R.N. on the children's unit tonight?"

Without any hesitation, Sylvia answered, "You are."

I felt a lump rise in my throat. "What? I'm the only nurse for our unit *and* for the children's unit?"

"Yeah, Haley called in sick, but don't worry 'cause Patrick and Tina and Janet will take care of the kids. They can handle it. Patrick can really run the whole unit on his own, except you'll have to do the meds since he's only a tech."

"How many kids?"

"Ten."

Then she added, as if repeating the words made it so, "But Patrick and Tina and Janet can handle it."

One of life's most important lessons is that sometimes you just have to do what you have to do. This was one of those situations. There simply was no other nurse available, and if I refused to take charge of the two units and walked out, there would be no nurse on our shift. If I refused, then either someone from the day shift would have to stay over and work a double shift or one of the supervisors or someone from administration would have to be called in. I'd probably be fired on top of it, so I figured I'd just have to hustle a little more than usual. It bothered me, though, because staffing was no where near adequate. Not for the numbers, nor for the acuity.

Tuesday. 4:20 p.m. Connie leaned over the counter and smiled. "Everything okay here? I'm leaving in a few minutes."

"You're kidding, right?" I asked. She looked at me quizzically, as if she didn't know what I was talking about, so I thought I'd better come straight out with it. "Connie, I'm the only nurse for both the adolescent and children's unit, and I only found out about it accidentally a few minutes ago. I wasn't told in report, and if I hadn't asked Sylvia about staffing directly, I probably still wouldn't know. It's usually a good idea to let the charge nurse know what she's in charge of."

She still looked confused, but then realization seemed to dawn and she drew in a deep breath. "I didn't know anything about this.

Nobody told me."

From her expression, I believed her. Connie had spent a number of years as a staff nurse at another facility prior to accepting the management position at Oak Haven, and she had a good understanding of the pressures of working on the units. Sometimes her support helped; sometimes it didn't.

Connie tried to be encouraging to the nursing staff but was often caught in a tug of war between the hospital administration and the unit staff. The desires and demands of the administration were not always in sync with the real-life needs of the staff and our patients.

Our conversation was interrupted by an overhead page calling me to the phone. It was the MHT who had escorted Nicole out for the X-ray.

"Debbi," she said breathlessly, "she ran away! She said she had to use the bathroom, and when my back was turned, she took off!"

Shit! I thought to myself. Out loud I asked, "Are you sure? Did you check everywhere?"

"Yes! I even looked outside, but she's gone. What should I do? Should I keep looking or what?"

"Well, if you've looked everywhere and you're sure she's gone, there's nothing else you can do there. Grab a cab and come back. We have a lot of people to call."

Connie was still at the counter, and I explained what had happened. "She's only fourteen, so I'll have to notify the police she's run away, right?"

"No, we don't have to do that anymore. Just let the administrator-on-call know, and he'll take care of notifying the police."

"So I don't have to call the police?" I liked to be absolutely clear about what I needed to do as well as what I should *not* do.

"Right. Just notify the doc and the administrator-on-call."

Tuesday. 5:00 p.m. Dr. Evans arrived on the same elevator as the MHT who had escorted Nicole to the other hospital, and I learned that she had already told him the gist of what had happened. I asked her to find out who the administrator-on-call was and to initiate a call to him while Evans and I talked. I was grateful to have that small amount of assistance, even though she told me

The Forgotten Future

she had to leave by 5:15.

Tuesday. 5:15 p.m. Caitlyn stepped into the office to tell me that she was gathering the kids for the community meeting.

"I'll be in as soon as I finish with Dr. Evans," I called after her. "Oh, and Caitlyn? Keep the kids on the unit for dinner tonight. We need to find out who knew about Nicole's plan to run and whether any of them know where she might go."

I turned to answer the ringing phone and spotted the three children's unit MHTs at the elevator with ten very noisy charges. "If you need help …" I threw up my hands. Patrick mirrored my *what-more-can-we-do?* gesture and ushered the boisterous crowd onto the elevator and headed to dinner.

A bordering-on-hysterical Brittany was on the phone. "Debbi, me and my mom got into a really big fight. She had me down on the floor and was hittin' me and stuff."

Timing is everything. I knew Brittany's situation with her mom had been troubled ever since her discharge, and now she had called the unit because she trusted and needed us. And because she thought we were the only ones who could help her. Unfortunately, I was caught in the evening's circumstances in which I was being pulled in a dozen different directions.

I leaned out the office door and looked across the hall through the group room's large reinforced glass window. The community meeting was loud, but Caitlyn appeared to have things under control. Maybe I could get through this conversation with Brittany quickly.

"Brittany, can you tell me what happened? Where are you now? Are you safe?" My biggest concern was that she might do something stupid, either out of desperation or to get back at her mom.

"She, um, was fightin' with her boyfriend, you know? And then I came into the room and she started screamin' that I was a tramp and was spyin' on them, and then Chuck, that's her boyfriend, got even more pissed at her and told her she was crazy, and he left. That's when she started hittin' me and pullin' my hair and stuff, so I hit her back. We were down on the floor, and I got up and ran over to my friend's house. That's where I am now."

Deborah Clark Ebel, R.N.

"Are you okay? Are you hurt?"

"Nah, I'm okay. I just don't know what to do." She was calmer, though still tearful. Her sniffling gave her away. "I was thinkin' about callin' my dad out in Ohio," she paused for a beat, and added, "but I don't know."

"Do you think he'll let you come out there? You know he wasn't willing to last time ..." The voices in the group room grew louder.

"I don't know. But then, um, my brother came here and said my mom said the Oak Grove people were comin' after me and were gonna make me go back there to stay. *For good.* Are you guys lookin' for me?"

"Brittany, I haven't heard anything about any of this and, no, we don't go out after people." I suspected her mom was up to her old tricks and was just trying to scare Brittany. The old men-in-the-white-coats ploy. It was working.

We continued talking for a few minutes until I felt the situation had eased and she had decided that she would call her dad. I also asked her to call me later in the evening, just to let me know what had happened and that she was safe.

The kids were angry and swearing as they filed out of the group room and were directed toward their rooms. Caitlyn stood in the hall encouraging the stragglers to continue straight on to their rooms rather than gather in the little cliques they so enjoyed and which could cause so many problems. I was glad Caitlyn and Barry were there, but I was angry about the unreasonable situation into which we had all been placed. Again. Not enough staff, neither from our perspective, nor for the kids' benefit or safety.

Caitlyn joined me in the nurses' office and leaned against the doorjamb. She unwrapped a piece of sugarless gum and popped it into her mouth. "A couple of them said they knew Nicole was going to run, but I think just about all of them knew. They said she had on three or four layers of clothes under her coat and money stuffed inside that bunny." She tilted her head and asked, "Unit shutdown?" already knowing the answer.

I nodded, knowing it could be a double-edged sword. On one hand, having the kids in their rooms where we could keep track of them was good. On the other hand, a shutdown might further aggravate the situation. Which was bad.

When a kid runs—AWOLs—from a psych unit, his or her plan to run is usually known by some, if not most, of their peers. Their friends keep the secret out of what they consider to be loyalty. The kids think that they have all the answers and don't understand the possible consequences of being alone and on the run. In some cases the runaway returns to a brutal or dangerous situation in which they sacrifice themselves in order to survive. Prostitution. Physical or sexual abuse. Drugs. They may engage in harmful behavior by accepting an offer of any sort of living situation with any type of person. They may even be suicidal.

Their friends on the unit think they're helping. The reality can be very different.

"Do you want me to start calling parents to let them know 'no visiting" because of the unit shutdown?" Caitlyn asked.

"We should, if there's time, but right now I'd rather have you keep an eye on the kids. A close eye." Priorities.

Caitlyn strode down the hall to take up her position with Barry at the end of the hall. I checked my watch and called the cafeteria for dinner trays. My shift would end in five-and-a-half hours.

Tuesday. 6:00 p.m. Nicole's parents had been divorced for almost three years when her mother found out that Nicole's dad had been sexually abusing her since she was a toddler. Since that time, Nicole had lived with her mom and rarely saw her father. She also had a history of running away.

Her mom was out of state on a business trip, and in her absence she had left Nicole in the care of her Uncle Tony. I dialed his number, and it rang three or four times before he picked up.

"Hello?"

"Hello, Mr. Ferguson? My name is Debbi, and I'm calling from Oak Haven Hospital."

Silence, and then, "Is Nicole causing problems already?"

"Well, not exactly, Mr. Ferguson. Nicole came in complaining of severe pain in her right hand, and this afternoon a member of our staff accompanied her over to Mercy Hospital Emergency Room for an X-Ray. Unfortunately, while they were there,

Deborah Clark Ebel, R.N.

Nicole ran away."

The next ninety seconds or so were filled with the angry rantings of a man who's had just about all he can stand and how he had told us she would run away and that we shouldn't have let her get into a situation where she could take off and he couldn't believe we were so incompetent as to allow her out of the hospital after he had warned us and that he thought she would go straight to her father and would do whatever she had to do to stay out of the hospital and continue to run with her friends and did I understand what he meant by doing whatever she had to do, etc., etc., etc.

He was right.

He asked if we had informed the police, and I told him that someone from the administration had taken care of that. He hung up on me.

Half an hour later he called back and angrily informed me that the police had never been notified and demanded that it be done immediately.

I apologized, all the while becoming more frustrated—for myself, for the kids, and for the parents who had expectations about the care their kids were receiving and which I knew they often were not. I told him that there was no excuse. There wasn't.

Immediately after Mr. Ferguson had his say, I telephoned the police and then called Mr. Ferguson back. Just before he hung up, he asked me to take a brief message for the hospital's chief administrator—that he would be at the hospital first thing in the morning and he expected some answers. Good ones.

Tuesday. 6:50 p.m. A loud crash got my attention, and Caitlyn and I raced down the hall toward the sound. The door to room 406 was closed, and I could hear pounding and kicking. I opened the door cautiously, calling out, "Abram? What's going on?"

His walls were splattered with stewed chicken and green beans, applesauce and cranberry juice. Abram paced the room like a caged animal.

"This shutdown sucks, man. You won't even let us go to the cafeteria to eat. You can't make us stay in our rooms like this. You're fuckin' out of your fuckin' minds." He picked up the desk chair and threw it against the wall for emphasis.

The Forgotten Future

I tried to get him to talk. He wouldn't. I asked him if he could promise me he would be safe and not cause any more damage if I let him stay in his room. He said, "Fuck no!" which I thought was pretty clear. I asked him to walk down to the seclusion room with me so he could calm down. Not a chance.

Although calling a Dr. Strong was the very last thing I wanted to do right then, I called it. I had no choice. Several of the staff members who arrived tried to talk Abram down, but he continued throwing things and threatening staff. There was no choice, and Abram was carried, kicking and screaming, swearing and threatening, amid jeers and heckles from the other kids, to the seclusion room where he was placed in four-points.

Tuesday. 7:30 p.m. "Debbi, you have a phone call." Caitlyn held the phone high in the air for me to see from down the hall.

"Who is it?" I asked as I hurried into the nurses' office. "Is it one of my sons? I really don't have time …"

"Nope, not this time. He didn't give his name, just started talking about a thirty-thousand-dollar bill for his daughter and then he asked for you. He sounded really pissed."

"A thirty-thousand-dollar bill? No name, huh?"

Caitlyn shook her head and shrugged.

I slipped into the desk chair, picked up the receiver, and pushed the flashing red button. "Hello," I said as cheerfully as I could manage, "this is Debbi."

It was Marci's dad. Marci was sixteen years old and had come in about a week previously after being arrested for stealing an ATM card from her best friend's mother's purse and then using it to withdraw several thousand dollars from the bank. In addition to the charges for the theft of the ATM card, Marci had half-a-page of other charges pending against her, including the theft of a couple of guns. She was into some pretty heavy stuff, including all kinds of drugs, and unless she made some radical changes, she would more than likely end up serving time in jail,

Her father had called several times over the course of the week, and I had put in a lot of time on the phone assuring him that Marci really needed help. He was totally unaware of many of the things that Marci had been doing and, unfortunately, I wasn't permitted to give him any information. Laws regarding confidentially and patients' rights prevented me from divulging any information about Marci's activities without her permission. She didn't want him to know what she had been up to, so our hands were tied. The most I could tell him was that she had been involved in some frankly dangerous activities and that unless things changed, she would probably end up in jail. Even saying that much was going out on a limb, but now he was feeling guilty about putting his "baby" into Oak Haven and was thinking about taking her out.

He needed frequent reassurance that he wasn't overreacting by having brought Marci to us. This phone call wasn't for reassurance, however. At least not directly.

"Debbi!" his voice boomed. He was angry, but didn't sound out of control. Yet. "I got this bill in the mail today. It's for thirty-thousand dollars! Marci's only been in there for seven days for Christ's sake!"

"Yeah, well, I can understand how you would be upset to get a bill for thirty-thousand dollars, but I don't know what to tell you. We really don't have anything to do with the billing or any of the charges up here on the unit. The business office takes care of all that." I paused, waiting for a comment or a response, but all I heard was silence, so I continued. "I'm not trying to put you off or anything, Mr. Broneil, but I really have no idea about the bill. What they've probably done is bill you in advance for her projected stay."

"Projected stay my ass!" he growled. "I'm taking out a goddam loan to pay for this fuckin' mess Marci has gotten herself into, and sending me a bill for thirty thousand dollars when she's only been in there for seven days really pisses me off." He paused and then threatened, "You know, maybe I should just come down there and get her right now and bring her home. I'm not sure Oak Haven is what she needs anyway."

Silently, I had to admit that I really wasn't sure that Oak Haven was the right place for Marci either. She wasn't doing anything in the hospital except bragging to the other kids about her exploits, and the group we had now admired and encouraged her.

The kids had too much free time during which they postured and bragged, schemed and plotted, and resisted any attempt to help them change their behaviors or attitudes. I didn't think Marci would be any different when she left Oak Haven from when she arrived, except that she might have a few new tricks in her bag.

"Mr. Broneil, I understand how upset you are, and you probably have every reason to be. I'm not going to do a sales job for Oak Haven Hospital. I know how much you love Marci, and I have to tell you once again that she has been engaged in some extremely serious and dangerous behaviors. She needs help, and if she doesn't get treatment here, then you absolutely must make sure she gets help somewhere else. You really cannot take her home and let her go back to doing the same things that she was doing."

I knew that Marci had been calling him every evening and telling him how much she hated the hospital and begging him to come get her and take her home. That would have been the worst thing he could do, so I kept talking. "I have three kids of my own, Mr. Broneil, and what I'm saying now is as much from a parent as from a professional. If you love your daughter as much as I believe you do, you *must* get her help."

I wanted to tell him about the guns and the sex parties and the fact that Marci had witnessed a girl being raped and thought it was "cool". I wanted to tell him that she had broken into houses with friends and stolen jewelry and electronic equipment, sold the items and bought drugs with the money. That she had stolen from friends and family as well as from strangers. That I really didn't think we were making any progress at all, nor would we in the remaining time that she would be with us and that her issues were probably going to require long-term care. But I couldn't. The law didn't allow me to say any of that, and even though I feared that her time at Oak Haven was probably a waste of time and money because she needed more than we could provide, I was worried that if her father discharged her prematurely, he would never be able to get her to go anywhere else.

We continued talking until I finally convinced him to get a good night's sleep and leave Marci in our care.

I hadn't given up yet and deep inside my soul there was still a very small glimmer of hope that maybe, just maybe, we might be able to make a difference.

Deborah Clark Ebel, R.N.

Tuesday. 8:00 p.m. I had to do a quick group on the children's unit. I would have half the kids, my choice which half, either the older or younger. I chose the older group, since at nine, ten, and eleven they were closer in age to those I was used to working with and wouldn't require a dramatic change in strategy or technique.

The group was one in which the kids are guided to talk about why they're in the hospital, what they had worked on that day, and how they were feeling about things in general. Sort of like a junior Wrap Up.

I quickly scanned the report sheet and gathered the kids together in the children's unit group room.

"Hi, guys, I'm Debbi." I smiled and looked around the circle. "Thanks for letting me sit in on your group. I usually work on the adolescent unit, but since there's no nurse on your unit tonight, I get to be with you for group."

There were several, "Oh yeahs" and "So *that's* where I've seen you before" and some other general chatter before we got started.

"Okay, how wants to start? Mary Lynn?"

"Yes. My name's Mary Lynn and my goal was to talk about my feelings about being molested." Mary Lynn was a sweet-faced nine-year-old who had been sexually molested by her dad. Since arriving on the unit, she had been overtly sexual toward every adult male—staff as well as visitors—that she could get close to. Things like stroking their thighs and kissing their necks.

"It's nice to meet you, Mary Lynn," I smiled. "Did you have a chance to talk about your feelings today?"

"Yeah, I talked in group this morning. I didn't like it when my dad molested me; I don't think parents should ever do that."

Several other kids murmured their agreement, and I said, "You're right, Mary Lynn. No adult should do things like that to any kid. Ever."

She offered a few more comments, and then I moved on. "Todd? Can you tell the group why you're here?" He sat with his knees drawn up to his chest.

No response. He wouldn't even look in my direction and just sat there, still and stone cold.

I waited.

The Forgotten Future

I waited some more.

"Todd? Is there anything you'd like to say?"

His glowering expression didn't change.

Todd was ten and had a serious problem controlling his anger. Before coming to the hospital, he had become angry at his mother and had used his father's hunting knife to stab her waterbed repeatedly, allowing gallons of water to flood the first-floor bedroom. Then he carved several filthy phrases into the headboard of her bed. Nothing would be accomplished by pushing him tonight, so we moved on to Eric.

"How are you doin' tonight, Eric? Was there something you were supposed to talk about today?"

Eric was eleven and had a chronically runny nose. Crusty. Gross. Before he came in, he had filled his baby sister's bottle with Scotch whisky and then fed it to her.

"I had to think of three positive ways to get my anger out without hurting anybody or anything."

"And did you?"

"Yeah. Number one, I can talk to my mom about what's making me mad. Number two, I can scream and yell into my pillow and hit it if I want to, and number three, I can go for a walk 'til I feel better."

"And did you already talk about this in group this morning?"

He nodded.

"That's great, Eric." It was getting late, and I wanted to wind things up quickly, so I moved on to Justin, an eleven-year-old new admission who smiled expectantly. "Welcome, Justin."

His smile was contagious.

"Do you feel comfortable enough to tell the group a little bit about yourself?"

"My name is Justin, and I molest little children." He looked around the group and grinned at everyone. They smiled back. It was obvious by his manner that he had done work in groups before.

"So, you have some problems you need to work on here in the hospital?"

"Yes. I molest little boys and little girls." He scanned the small group again, still smiling and sounding like a politician after the vote. "There was Jeffrey and David, and once when I visited little Amanda, I ..."

"Sounds like you have a lot of things to work on while you're here." I cut across him, not because of the topic, but because I didn't think we needed a litany of his victims and activities. Not tonight. It was getting late, and I couldn't afford to become embroiled in anything too heavy. Besides, he was too eager to share.

"Yeah, I do. Don't you want to hear what I did to little Amanda?" he continued. "I ..."

"Justin," I said firmly but not unkindly. "I think your clinician will be pleased you're so willing to talk in group, but I'm afraid you'll have to wait until tomorrow to tell us anymore. I have to get back to the teenagers now," I looked at the clock, "and I think it's time for you guys to get ready for bed, isn't it?"

It was, and they did. I returned to the adolescent unit, reminding myself that society's problems start early.

The remainder of the evening flew, with passing meds, checking in with each of the kids to see if they were doing their assignments, running to the hospital pharmacy to get a med that should have been available on the unit but wasn't, answering the phone, completing various reports, monitoring the kids in the seclusion room, charting on each patient, and the myriad of other details that kept cropping up.

When I finally took a break, I realized how tired and hungry I was. I hadn't eaten since lunch and the cafeteria had long ago closed, so I checked out the patient kitchen. My dinner? A glass of watered-down lemonade and several packages of Oak Haven saltines. I felt no guilt.

*   *   *   *

Connie Kincaid and Dr. Carmichael called a staff meeting to "discuss issues impacting on the efficient operation of the adolescent unit". Those of us actually working with the patients thought we knew what to expect, but as usual we were surprised.

Dr. Carmichael had some new ideas he wanted to try out, ideas to give the kids "more freedom and more time to do what they want". Based on reports from the kids, he felt staff—particularly evening staff—were too strict and didn't "let the kids just be kids and enjoy themselves". He had requested that the administration have cable TV hooked up so the kids could watch television at night. He also wanted us to hold fewer groups in the evening and allow later bedtimes for everyone. "And how about allowing cell phones in the evening?" he asked. He kept talking about wanting the kids to have "fun".

Another idea of his was to do away with the point system we used to award levels and privileges. "Everyone," he said, "should be equal."

The fact was, we rarely had any groups in the evening anymore. Those we did have were mostly ones that had previously been done by contract therapists to whom the hospital had to pay an hourly rate. Now those groups were part off the nursing staff's responsibilities. Unfortunately, with such high acuity and frequently inadequate staffing, more often than not the groups fell by the wayside as we dealt with more urgent situations.

We took the kids to the gym for "rec" almost every evening, and they watched far too many entertainment videos. The kids, in *our* view, already had more free time than was judicious. Since we had the kids for only a very brief time due to insurance-driven shortened hospital stays, the unit staff felt we should utilize the time for the benefit of the kids—not spend time entertaining them. They could watch *Grey's Anatomy* at home.

As for the "point" system: points and levels were an incentive the kids would work for. A young person who couldn't care less about working on his attitude toward authority would most definitely work to get a higher level which would allow him to make more phone calls or have friends in to visit.

I think Dr. Carmichael said it best when he announced that when we implemented his new plans, Oak Haven would have a "pointless" program.

*   *   *   *

Deborah Clark Ebel, R.N.

The next afternoon, Howard caught up with me as I walked the halls to do first rounds. "So, did you see the restraints Tyrone chewed through?" he asked, almost too casually.

I stepped into the group room and did a quick head count before answering. Back in the hall, we continued walking. I smiled and wondered what the punch line would be. "Howard, what are you talking about? Chewed through?"

"Yes! They had some problems with him last night and they had to put him in four-points. He chewed through both wrist restraints!"

"Get out of here. That's impossible."

"Debbi, I tell you ..."

"Howard, the straps are an inch wide and probably almost a quarter-inch thick. They're *leather,* for god's sake."

He had been waiting for my reaction and grabbed my arm to lead me toward the resource room. He fumbled with his keys and unlocked the door, ushering me in. "Over there." He had an I-told-you-so grin as he motioned toward a pair of leather wrist restraints on the far table.

I picked up one of the restraints and turned it over in my hands. I could see where it had been chewed through, as well as where the leather was stained from Tyrone's saliva. "Oh m'god! Look at this!" I looked from my hands to Howard, then back to my hands. "How long did it take him to chew through these, anyway?"

"Who knows? Night staff went into the seclusion room early this morning and found him sitting up on the bed. His biggest complaint was about the taste."

"They hadn't done rounds during the night?" I asked, incredulously.

"They said they watched him on the monitor."

Yeah. Right. But these chewed restraints meant that they hadn't actually seen him for whatever period of time it had taken him to chew through two leather straps. The possibilities of what might have happened gave me chills.

*   *   *   *

The Forgotten Future

It seemed like Ryan and I clashed over everything. I set limits, and he pushed them. I enforced a consequence, and in Ryan's eyes I became an unreasonable ogre. Oak Haven's own Nurse Ratched.

Still, I sensed something there, something intangible that, despite his antagonism and profanity, made me believe that there might be a chance that he wanted to overcome the devastation of his childhood enough to do some work.

My first inkling that I might be right came when I didn't expect it. Ryan and I had locked horns once again over something relatively inconsequential, and he had stormed off to his room, swearing.

I gave him a few minutes and then decided I would go down and clear things up. I tapped lightly on his door. "Ryan? This is Debbi. We need to talk."

I heard him grunt something that I took to be assent, so I walked into his room and found him sitting on his bed. He'd done absolutely no work on his issues since coming to Oak Haven, yet he was a bright kid. I believed that he was a kid who, *if he wanted to,* could *do* and *be* and *become.* He could achieve and accomplish, but if he didn't do an about-face soon ... This was one of those times when I thought a kid might need a little extra push in the right direction. I hoped I was right.

"Ryan, I think we need to get a few things straightened out here." Although he had a history of violence, I wasn't frightened, nor even nervous, as I leaned against the desk. I was, however, cautious and, although I plowed ahead, I watched him carefully for any sudden or unexpected movement. I also left plenty of space between us.

I didn't know Ryan well enough to be able to predict with any certainty how he might react to my blunt confrontation. I *thought* I knew, but he was still somewhat of an unknown. "You're here in this hospital whether you want to be or not, and you can put in your time doing nothing, just like you've been doing, or you can spend some time trying to work out what has been, up until now, a pretty lousy deal."

He was listening, which was something.

"I know it's been lousy. It's been shitty and it's been hell. It sucks. But you can't change what's already happened; you can only choose what the rest of your life is going to be." I was angry, not at Ryan, but at his father and at every single person who has ever dared hurt a child like Ryan had been hurt. I was angry at a society that tolerates the abuse of kids like Ryan and all the others. I was frustrated by the lack of intense outrage toward situations that turn so many of our kids into angry souls who lash out at others and hurt people before they, themselves, are hurt again. And I was saddened by my inability to do more.

"You can choose to just continue on the way you have been going and keep hangin' with the gangs and the drugs and blaming the rest of the world for everything bad that's ever happened to you. You can keep up the tough guy bullshit, or you can decide to work hard as hell to make things better for yourself." I sighed and glanced around the room. My mouth was dry and my throat was tight. He hadn't told me to eat shit and die yet, so maybe we were getting somewhere.

Ryan stood at the window, gazing out at the distance. I bowed my head for a minute or so, and we stood there. Silent. I reminded myself that I was starting to care too much once again, and that this could be a tough one if I let it. But I just hated it when there was so much possibility in a kid and it was lost. I closed my eyes and shook my head from side to side, thinking, I just hate it …

"Ryan?" I lifted my head and looked straight at him, speaking softly now. "I'm not here to give you a hard time. You can hate me if you want, or you can think I'm the worst person in the world." I tilted my head to the side and grinned, "Hell, you can even call me a bitch if you want … trust me … I've been called *much* worse things." I could see his smile reflected in the window.

"Look, I'm willing to work on this thing with you, but we've got to have an understanding and some ground rules. It's not gonna be easy and it's not gonna be fun. But I'm going to be here whether you work or not. I just think you have to give it a chance. Give yourself a chance. I'm not your enemy."

He turned and looked at me without speaking.

"Deal?" I said.

He nodded. "How do I start?"

The Forgotten Future

We talked for a long time that evening. It was as if the dam had burst and things just started spilling out. He told me about how when he was little his dad would go out and party and then come home drunk or stoned. Ryan always prayed his dad would be in a good mood so he wouldn't get hit. Or worse.

And if he was in a bad mood?

"He'd throw things at me, kick me, give me black eyes and bruises all over my body. A couple of times he even whipped me with a bullwhip. Real leather. Or he'd make me go out to the wood pile to pick out a piece of wood that I wanted to get beat with."

"Sometimes he'd ask me to help him with something and I was so nervous because he'd tell me to hand him a tool or hold on to something. I would do the wrong thing on accident and he would hit me for it. Once he asked me to plug the vacuum in one socket, and I plugged it in a different socket and he started screaming and beat me with the vacuum cord."

Then, of course, there was the sexual abuse we'd heard about when he was admitted.

"You know, I've never talked to anybody like this before." He thought for a moment, then, "When I was a kid in school I was always a clown. I always wanted to make people laugh. I made everybody laugh, even the teacher, except for this one girl. She never laughed at me and I couldn't figure out why until this one day we were walking home from school and I was trying to make her laugh and she wouldn't. *She just wouldn't.*" He looked at me straight on. "You know what she said to me?"

"No." I shook my head.

"She told me, 'You don't have to be like this, Ryan.'" He looked away briefly, then back at me. "I never spoke to her again."

"She knew. She knew what you were doing, Ryan."

"Yeah. Now I guess I know, too."

I believe he did.

Chapter 9
Troubles Never-Ending

"**R**ec" time was usually a treat. The kids would run and jump and scream and yell and work off pent-up energy.

And anger.

Somersaults. Table games. Pool. Exercise bikes. Basketball.

BASKETBALL! They loved it! The fifty-inch fourteen-year-old teamed with the six-foot-one twelve-year-old.

Sometimes I would get so caught up watching them that for a few minutes I could forget where I was and who the kids were and what their lives and histories were. With music blaring, they ran and sweated and competed and worked together. Hair flying, their feet barely touched the ground. I marveled at their freedom and their joy in playing. They were *having fun,* like kids should.

The African-American kid and the Latino, the white and the Native American, the Asian and the middle Eastern, the kid from Chicago and the one from West Virginia, the boy and the girl, the short, tall, heavy, slight, bright and not-quite-so-bright, the one who played the bagpipes and the one who played the boom box, laughing and squealing 'til it was hard to remember where they were, and for a short while the horrors of their lives receded into the mist.

I felt like I could watch them forever during those times. I could imagine we were outside on a soft summer evening, playing on

Deborah Clark Ebel, R.N.

some neighborhood court. The maple and gum trees swaying with the breeze while proud mothers and fathers watched the game, shouting encouragement to their kids. Younger children imitated their older siblings, and the occasional dog ran onto the court, disrupting play momentarily. I wanted those times to never end.

And then back to reality. It might be an elbow into someone's ribs or an overly aggressive charge toward another player. It might only be that rec time was up. Whatever the reason, we would return to the unit, and the kids would return to the realities of their lives.

I hope that somewhere in America the game continues …

*   *   *   *

Nick's father had stood him up again. In the weeks Nick had been with us, his father had repeatedly made plans to pick up his son for a pass and then would be a no-show.

Nick had been a real surprise for all of us, for despite the trepidation with which we had met his admission, he had turned out to be a really good kid. The only time we ever saw him angry was when his father let him down which, unfortunately, was every time he had contact with him. It was at those times that his sadness and loneliness and disappointment were expressed as anger.

Gradually, and with a lot of support from staff, he became stronger and better able to understand that his father's rejection and neglect of him were not his fault. Rather, his father simply was incapable of being a parent, never mind a good parent.

Nick was a good-looking young man who was always neat and clean. He took pride in his appearance, not in a vain way, but in that he always presented himself well. Over his weeks in the hospital, his hair grew long, way too long, and he began to feel embarrassed by his appearance. Two or three weeks previously, he had begun lobbying his father to take him for a haircut, and this was the day his father had promised.

Having grown accustomed to being blown-off by his dad, Nick seemed more disappointed about missing the haircut than about not having a visitor. He was scheduled for an interview for residential placement in a few days, and he wanted to look his best.

The Forgotten Future

By the time he asked us for help, we had already begun working on it. The nurses and MHTs pitched in a few bucks apiece, and Caitlyn agreed to take him out for the haircut. Nick was delighted. What he didn't know, though, was that we had also chipped in enough to buy him a new pair of jeans and a shirt. His new interview outfit. And then we gave Caitlyn explicit instructions: she was not to bring Nick back to the hospital until they had stopped and had their fill of pizza at the local pizzeria. He was going to have fun on his pass if *we* had anything to do with it!

* * * *

Friday. 3:00 p.m. We had thirteen kids on the unit, including two in the seclusion room and three on special programs who required close monitoring. We were once again staffed with only three people—Howard, Caitlyn, and me—and I was scheduled to do a program that would take me away from the open unit and from a majority of the kids. That couldn't possibly be done, and once again I had to cancel a group.

We learned that the drug and alcohol group leader was ill, so there would be no drug ed group, either. All the kids had been confined to the unit for lunch because of negative behavior and had been told that we would reassess the situation regarding dinner.

Howard and I talked, and we decided we would lay out very clear expectations in order to try to avoid hassles later in the shift. No one wanted any problems.

With this in mind, I made rounds and did a short one-to-one with each of the kids, being very specific regarding assignments to be done and behavioral expectations. One girl requested ibuprofen for cramps, and a couple needed their pencils sharpened. No problems so far.

Friday. 5:00 p.m. I sat in on the community meeting while Howard took a dinner break. All in all, the meeting went poorly. The kids were at each other's throats. Some had legitimate complaints; some were just scapegoating. Most were just plain instigating. My presence in the meeting rapidly went from that of an observer/advisor, to mediator, to disciplinarian.

I ejected one of the boys from the meeting for making inappro-priate sexual comments and another for glorifying drug use. They each had to sit on the time-out bench in the hall for five minutes. Quietly. Of course, that meant I had to stand in the doorway of the group room so I could watch them while I continued to participate in the community meeting.

Friday. 5:30 p.m. I quickly passed both my 5:00 and 6:00 meds and made the decision that Howard and Caitlyn would take most of the kids down to the cafeteria for dinner. The kids had been up on the unit all day and were beginning to show signs of cabin fever. They could probably use a change of scenery.

I explained to William, Tyrone, and April that, because of their negative behavior, they would have dinner on the unit and in their rooms.

"You can't keep me up here!" declared William. "I've been up here for twenty-four hours straight and I should be able to go to the cafeteria to eat." He started through the door, but Howard stepped in front of him.

"William!" bellowed Howard. "Don't start!"

"Fuck you! Get outta my way!"

"C'mon man. It's no big deal," said Tyrone.

"He's right, William. They're not gonna let you go, so you might as well just stay up here with us." That was from April.

For whatever reason, William listened to what they said. He gave the wall a kick, gave Howard and me the finger and said, "screw you, fuckheads". Then he turned and swaggered down the hall toward his room.

Howard and I exchanged glances in which he asked, "Will you be okay?" and to which I nodded "hope so", and he and Caitlyn moved the ones going to the cafeteria toward the elevator.

Friday. 5:45 p.m. The three kids remaining on the unit shouted obscenities and sexual comments back and forth across the hall. They slammed doors shut, then opened them up and slammed them shut again.

I passed out dinner trays and reminded them that they were supposed to be quiet and in their rooms, but they knew as well as I that there was nothing I could do to enforce what I was saying.

The Forgotten Future

"Bite me!" was probably the kindest comment I heard.

Friday. 5:50 p.m. The "ding" of the elevator caught my attention. I was hoping it might be Howard and Caitlyn returning from the cafeteria, but I knew it was too soon. The elevator door opened, and Patrick from the children's unit arrived with a kicking and screaming nine-year-old named James.

James practically lived at Oak Haven, having been with us six or seven times. He was a big, stocky kid, weighing in at a little over ninety pounds. Every evening he threw one of his fits and invariably ended up spending time in the seclusion room, kicking the door, pounding the floor, and screaming. If there was sufficient staff, that wasn't a problem.

Tonight, though, there was no one else available to help, and I watched Patrick try every tactic he knew in an attempt to convince James to exit the elevator. He coaxed and cajoled, but James would have none of it. James stood in the back corner of the elevator, swearing, and refusing to move. "You can't fuckin' make me do nothin'," he said, "and I'll kick your ass if you try."

Nobody could say Patrick didn't try.

I stood at the nurses' office door watching the elevator, watching my hallway, hoping James would cooperate. Wishing Howard would return from the cafeteria.

"Debbi, could you give me a hand here?" Patrick asked sharply.

I hesitated, wondering and hedging my bets about whether I dared turn my back on my three kids for the short time it would take to move James into the back area. I really didn't have a choice because James had to be moved and there was no one else to help Patrick. Taking one last peek down the hall, I walked out of the office and around to the elevator.

I sneaked glances into the adolescent unit hall while we were at the elevator, and I didn't like what I saw. While we were in the back area putting James into the seclusion room, I didn't like what I heard either. Fortunately, just as we finished up with James, Howard and Caitlyn arrived with the rest of the adolescents. Those adolescents who had visitors began their visits, and those who didn't started playing games or disappeared into their rooms.

Friday. 7:45 p.m. "Fuckin bitch! I'm gonna kill you!" Kevin's heartfelt profanity was followed by a kick to his door and several other unintelligible mutterings. He stormed toward the far end of the hall, smashing his fist into the wall several times along the way.

"Uh, oh, we got a problem." I raced down the hall with Howard close on my heels.

Kevin was still shouting when he barged into April's room. "Where the fuck are you, April?" He opened her bathroom door and, seeing the room was empty, slammed the door with a loud bang.

"Kevin! What's going on?" Howard demanded.

"Look at this!" Kevin screamed, shoving a red soggy mess in front of our faces. "Bitch cunt April left this in my door!" He threw the mass on the floor and continued pacing and cursing.

I stooped to look and realized that it was a wet, bloody tampon. Kevin and April had been at each other's throats for the past week, but if she had really put this at his door, she had passed beyond any reasonable or acceptable boundary.

Howard stood in front of Kevin, speaking softly and just letting him get things off his chest. Kevin was gradually calming, so maybe we would be able to ease the situation and avoid any further problems.

I slipped on a pair of gloves and picked up the tampon. I took it into April's bathroom for closer inspection. In the brighter light it was obvious it wasn't a *bloody* tampon, but rather a *ketchupy* one. Ketchup had been smeared on a wet tampon to give the appearance of blood, so it wasn't quite as gross as it first appeared. Nevertheless, it was a crude and ignorant thing to do. I wrapped the tampon tightly inside paper towels and went in search of April.

I found her in the community room and invited her to join me in one of the conference rooms. Now, please! She winced when I opened the paper towels to show her the contents, but I thought I caught the slightest hint of a smirk. "You know anything about this?" I asked, holding out the tampon for her to see.

"O-o-o gross! That's *nasty*!" she squealed. She covered her face with both hands while bending and squatting to show her disgust. "Who would do something like that?"

"I was hoping you could tell me," I replied. "Kevin found this in his door, and I thought you might know something about it."

"Me? No way. That's too sick. Whooooo!" She could hardly contain her enjoyment of the situation, but she wasn't going to budge in her denial.

After going back-and-forth with her for a while, I finally gave up. There was no way she was going to admit planting the tampon, if, indeed, she was the one. When Howard and I discussed it later, he told me that Kevin was positive that it was April because she had threatened to get even with him for "breaking up" with her. Unfortunately, without anyone on the unit willing to step forward, it was his word against hers.

Friday. 10:30 p.m. With rec, charting, a couple of one-to-ones, snack, and medications, we somehow made it through most of the evening without a major disaster. I saw Howard go into the media room and turn on the local news. "Howard, I'm going to be in the resource room taping report, so can you come out and keep an eye on the hall?"

He glanced up and said, "Yeah, sure," and returned to the news.

The Kardex and report papers lay out in front of me. I turned on our new tape recorder and began. "Hi, this is Debbi reporting for the three to eleven-thirty shift for Friday evening. We have thirteen kids on the unit, with three on special programs."

"The unit has been tough tonight … the kids are negative and testing limits, but I'll get into that in a minute. In room 401A you have Nick T. He's fourteen, Dr. Carmichael's patient, in with a diagnosis of oppositional …"

I hit the pause button on the recorder and looked toward the small window in the door. I thought I had heard someone tapping on the door. Maybe Howard needed me. The hall was dark, so I couldn't see through the window. Believing it was Howard, I motioned for him to come in. "It's okay," I said.

I waited, and then, figuring I was mistaken, I turned on the recorder and began speaking again. "Nick's in with oppositional defiant disorder. He's had a really good evening, didn't feed into the negativity on the …"

There it was again. I stood and walked to the door. Pressing my nose against the glass, I peered into the dark hallway. No Howard. I knew I had heard something, so I opened the door quietly, holding pressure on the doorknob.

I squinted up and down the dim passage. Everything seemed as it should. No sound and nothing out of place. Taking a step backward, I was just about to shut the door when I glanced at the floor behind the door.

Tyrone!

"Where do you think you're going?"

He remained crouched for a moment, surprised to have been discovered. As my eyes adjusted to the shadowy hallway, I saw that he was dressed for the outdoors—heavy winter coveralls and jacket, knitted cap and gloves. Pulling himself to his full height, he frowned, as if calculating how formidable a resistance I might be.

He apparently figured *not much*, because he sneered and slowly began to saunter toward the exit.

"Howard! I need help ... now!" I yelled. I hoped he was still in the media room, which was between me and the elevator. I knew I was certainly no match for Tyrone, so the best I could do was to lock the outer door. Rushing into the nurses' office, I threw the switch just as a bewildered Howard appeared.

Howard directed a questioning glance toward Tyrone and then at me.

"I was taping report when I heard a noise. When I came out, I found our friend here, dressed for the outdoors and crawling along the floor."

"Guess he doesn't like it here." Howard turned to Tyrone. "Okay, Tyrone, let's take a walk."

Tyrone was a big guy, but Howard was bigger. That night Tyrone didn't push his luck and returned to his room without a struggle. We took his outdoor wear away from him for the remainder of his stay. Just in case.

The next day, Tyrone explained to the day shift that he was thirsty and had simply gone into the hall "looking for juice" when we jumped him for no reason. Looking for juice? On the floor? Nice try, Tyrone.

*   *   *   *

The Forgotten Future

I was in Tabitha's room engaged in a pretty heavy session when I heard a loud *crash*. Caitlyn was monitoring the hall, so I knew she would check it out. When I heard her screams, though, I raced toward her cries.

Nick's room was dark, but I could see two figures struggling near the window. Caitlyn was a big woman, but sometimes even that was no match against the strength of a young, physically-healthy male. They were both yelling, but I couldn't make out what either was saying.

I rushed forward to join them as Caitlyn cried, "The light bulb! He still has the light bulb!" I hesitated only seconds, trying to figure out what was happening, where to look, what to do.

"I've got him! He has a broken light bulb! In his hand!"

Then I understood. His blood-soaked right hand clinched the remnants of a broken light bulb. I tried to pry his fingers loose, but he resisted and pulled his fingers into a tight fist. He cried out in pain.

"Nick, honey, it's gonna be okay," I said gently. "Nick, you just need to loosen your fingers a little. That's it. Okay, good. Just a little more …"

As I opened his hand, I could see the slivers of glass and metal and filament wire, gooey with blood. I grabbed a washcloth from the end of the bed and gently wiped the foreign material from his hand. I placed the cloth over what had become a bloody mess.

"His left arm, too," Caitlyn said breathlessly as she began to loosen her hold. "He was cutting his wrist when I came in."

He was no longer resisting, just moaning softly. My heart sank as I reached over and pulled his arm from his side. More blood. The towel from the bed found its place on his arm.

While we waited for medical assistance to arrive, Nick haltingly tried to explain what had happened. Everything had been going well all day, and he was listening to his iPod. The last song he heard was *Cat's In The Cradle*, a mournful ballad about a father who never had time for his son. A tale about a boy who grew up to be just like his father. A song that Nick saw as reflective of his own life. He reached into his desk lamp, unscrewed the light bulb, broke it, and cut his wrist.

Deborah Clark Ebel, R.N.

He sat on the end of his bed crying as if his heart was breaking. Mine was.

* * * *

Texas was seventeen and had been living on the streets for two years. She'd seen her mom only a few times during that time. I met her mom once, when she visited Texas and dropped off some too-small clothes.

Her mom was young. Texas said she was thirty-one, but she looked fiftyish. Not a good fifty. A lined, worn, ashen fifty.

Texas dressed country, listened to Kenny Chesney and the Dixie Chicks, and had affected a southwestern twang. She didn't think she had anything in common with other kids her age and, in fact, most kids didn't care for her. She was shy and standoffish and construed their indifference toward her as malignment of her "country" ways.

She liked to hang around the nurses' office, running errands, getting supplies, even sharpening pencils. Snippets of conversation were all that she would give us. She said she could write her thoughts easier than speak them and asked me to read her journal. The journal told how her father left before she was born, her mother and first stepfather divorced when she was four, and her uncle molested her whenever she visited him.

When she was six, her new stepfather started molesting her.

When she was eight, a neighborhood boy tried to rape her.

At thirteen, her grandfather wrestled with her and rubbed lotion on her body under her clothing.

From fourteen to fifteen her mother's live-in boyfriend physically and emotionally abused her. He called her slut, whore, cocksucker, dyke, and any other names he could think of and mocked her about "sleeping" with her stepfather, uncle, and grandfather. He threw her out of the house and told her not to return.

The next two years were spent on the streets or in shelters, moving from guy to guy, bottle to bottle, and drug to drug.

She didn't believe her life could ever be any different.

The Forgotten Future

I wondered. Could it? Could it ever be any different?

*   *   *   *

The crisis workers were both busy with other clients, so the hospital operator called me. With eighteen kids—including three on full AWOL precautions—and a brand-new mental health tech in training, I really didn't have time to talk on the phone, but Jane said the woman was crying and I was the only one available to talk to her. "Hang up," directed Jane, "and I'll put her through."

I grabbed the pink telephone intake form and picked up on the first ring. "Adolescent unit, this is Debbi," I said in my most professional telephone voice.

"I think I need some help with my daughter. I think she may need to come and stay at your hospital for a while?" Her voice went up and sounded like a question.

"Okay, we'll see what we can do. Would you tell me how old your daughter is?"

"She's fourteen." Sigh. "Lately she's been lying to me about where she's going and what she's doing … her grades are going down … I just don't know what to do …"

"You say she's lying? Are we talking about once or twice or a lot?"

"Almost every day. Almost every day she's lying about something."

"Okay, I understand. So, what happened today that has you so upset that you decided to call Oak Haven?"

"See … she was over her friend's house, and she called me at work and said her and her friend and her friend's mother were going to the mall. I don't let her hang out at the mall like a lot of kids, so I said, are you sure Trish's mother is taking you, and she said yes."

"Okay … and then what?"

"Well, then I found out they took the bus and Trish's mom didn't go! She didn't even know she was supposed to take them," she said indignantly.

"Uh, huh. They lied to you and took the bus to the mall?" I

continued making notes, waiting for the other shoe to fall. "And then?"

"Well, that's just it! She wasn't supposed to take the bus; she was supposed to go with a parent."

I put my pen down on the desk. My eyes were tired, and I rubbed them with my now-free hand. Surely there was more to this that a one-time bus ride to the mall. "All right, let me ask you some more questions. How about curfews? Is she staying out late or not coming home?"

"No ... she always comes home when she's supposed to."

"How about alcohol? Is she drinking or using any drugs that you're aware of? Pot?"

"Well, I know she was drinking some a few months ago ... pot? I don't know ... she might've tried it. I don't know. I don't think so ... I don't know."

"Do the two of you fight a lot? Not just arguing, but is there any physical fighting?" I rested my forehead on my hand.

"Not really. We get along pretty good most of the time. It's just that she tells lies and some of her friends are not the best."

"So basically, you're mostly concerned about her telling lies and about her friends. And some drinking, but you don't know how much. Is that right?"

"Yes. I just don't know what to do with her anymore."

I felt sorry for the woman because she sounded so distraught over what was minor compared to what we were used to dealing with. My guess was that what she and her daughter both needed was a reminder of their respective roles. What she didn't need, in my opinion, was to place her daughter in a psychiatric hospital. I asked the last, very bottom-line question. "Do you feel either your daughter or anyone else is at any risk of harm tonight? Do you feel safe having her at home until you can speak with someone tomorrow?"

"Yeah, I guess we'll be okay. Yeah. Yeah, she's okay, just watching television right now."

I gave her instructions to call the crisis worker in the morning and request an appointment for outpatient counseling. Maybe this would turn out to be one of those times when the parent got some guidance before things got out of hand. I wished her luck.

*   *   *   *

Hannah was fifteen, and since the age of nine, she had spent much of her time in institutions of one type or another. She had been living back at home now for almost two years.

Her mother had recently surprised the family with two declarations: she was divorcing her husband of twenty-six years, and she and Hannah would be residing with mom's new female partner, Lori. Needless to say, both announcements were upsetting to Hannah. She didn't understand the breakup of her family, and, while she had been aware of her mother's bisexuality for quite some time, she had never expected it to seriously impact their—her –way of life.

Hannah and her mom moved into Lori's expensive two-bedroom apartment and things took a dramatic turn for the worse. Chronically oppositional, Hannah became assaultive toward both her mother and Lori and resumed her former runaway behavior. Most recently, she had been suspended after assaulting a teacher at her small, rural high school.

Hannah looked young for her age. She was probably only five-foot-one or so and had straight, stringy, shoulder-length hair of a non-descript color. Coke-bottle-thick tortoiseshell glasses made her eyeballs appear about to bulge out past the lenses. She breathed heavily through an open mouth, giving a slight wheeze with each expiration.

Her history included having been molested by an uncle when she was about six, yet, despite years of therapy and multiple hospitalizations, she had not fully recovered. She had been an inpatient at Oak Haven five years previously, and a doctor's written comparison of the psych testing done at that time with testing done on this admission found, "a young lady of fifteen who sounds exactly the same as she did at ten. She is extremely overactive, anxious, tangential, impulsive and careless. Distractible throughout the session, with the exception of very short periods where she became serious and was able to focus on the task."

The report went on to describe "much confusion about sexuality and being over stimulated by the topic in general". Interestingly, one of her recent issues was her frequent sexual activity with younger boys. Boys of ten and eleven.

Well, I wasn't sure how effective we would be at addressing her issues, but we would surely try.

*   *   *   *

The medical report gave the full details of what damage was done when Timothy put the pistol to his head. He had used a carbon dioxide pellet gun, a type of "fun" gun many think of as relatively harmless. After he pulled the trigger, the pellet penetrated his right temporal lobe, passed into the region of the basal nuclei in the left temporal lobe, ricocheted off the inside of the skull, and finally lodged in the left temporal cortex.

Dr. Trudel had made arrangements to transfer Timothy to a large medical center in the South that specialized in neurological injuries. Timothy would leave in just a few days and, while he could be a royal pain in the neck and had to be watched constantly, I would miss him. In many ways he was just an innocent little boy.

"Debbi?"

I was surprised to see Timothy at the nurses' office door. "Yes, sir. What can I do for you?"

"What's your last name?" He held a pencil and a torn piece of paper.

"Ebel. E-B-E-L."

He wrote slowly.

"That's right ... E—B ..."

"E—B—E—L?"

"Right." I watched as he sprinted back down the hall to his room.

He returned a few minutes later, smiling and holding something behind his back. "Debbi Ebel?"

"Yes, Timothy ..." I swiveled around in my chair to face him. "Whatcha got?"

The Forgotten Future

"It's for you." He held out a piece of paper. "I made this for you."

It was a piece of lined notebook paper on which he had drawn and colored a big, red heart. Right in the middle, he had written, "Debbi Ebel", and underneath, "From Timothy".

"It's so you'll never forget me." He flashed that beautiful smile once more.

I reached out and hugged him, thinking *not a chance, Timothy. Not a chance.*

*   *   *   *

"Hannah! Come out of the office *now!*" Caitlyn rarely bellowed, but when she did, it carried to the far end of the hall.

I exited the group room to see if she needed help and found there were already a couple of staff people standing by. Waiting.

Hannah stood in the nurses' office, surrounded by papers and charts that she had thrown to the floor. She hurriedly punched numbers into the wall phone, but was so agitated she misdialed several times and had to redial. All the while, Caitlyn continued insisting she hang up the phone and come out of the office.

Hannah refused. "No! Leave me alone. I can't dial the phone with you fuckin' runnin' your mouth!" She took another swipe at the desk and toppled the pencil sharpener and file tray. She glared at Caitlyn.

Expecting that sooner or later we'd need an order for something or other to help calm Hannah, I figured I'd go ahead and call the doctor. I gave Hannah a wide berth, but otherwise ignored her as I walked past to the phone on the other end of the nurses' office. She looked at me briefly, but Caitlyn must have seemed more of an immediate threat, and she refocused her attention.

I've never been exactly clear about what happened next. Or why.

Hannah was screaming into the phone, "Come get me!" and I was speaking to Dr. Evans. Barry ran in and grabbed Hannah from behind. He held her in a big bear hug and dragged her out into the hall. "Can I get some help here?" he yelled. There was no organization, no game plan. No one had called the takedown.

Barry had backed into a corner, his arms clasped around Hannah's upper arms and chest. Hannah wriggled and kicked and was slipping downward from his grasp. She pulled up her right leg and donkey-kicked Barry. "Goddammit! Somebody get her legs!" he barked.

Staff stood looking on, seeming unsure how to react since this was not a coordinated effort. Caitlyn snapped to attention first and rushed forward to help.

I hung up the phone and started out into the hall. I knew what was coming even as it unfolded. It was one of those I-see-it-happening-but-I-don't-believe-it-deja-vu-I-just-can't-move-fast-enough events.

Caitlyn leaned forward to restrain Hannah's legs just as Hannah pulled back and flung her foot full-force into Caitlyn's face. There was a deafening *thwack!* as Caitlyn crumbled to the floor.

I heard someone scream, "Oh my god!" and saw the rest of the staff move in. I ran and knelt beside Caitlyn. Blood gushed from her nose and lip. Disoriented, she was conscious but looked like she didn't know where she was or why. Hannah still kicked and swore.

"Get her out of here. Just get her out of here!" I screamed at the others.

I looked up and saw a couple of the kids peeking out of their room. "Girls? Can I get some towels? Quickly?" I leaned over and gently rubbed Caitlyn's shoulders. She whimpered softly, and the carpet turned crimson.

She was four months pregnant.

*　　*　　*　　*

It was my day off, but I had agreed to come in and do a half-shift with an adult unit patient. Coming in at 3:00 in the afternoon, I was looking forward to leaving at 7:30 and spending the rest of the evening with my family. I should have known better.

At 7:15, as I was giving report to the incoming adult unit nurse, I received a call from Jackie up on the fourth floor. "Debbi?

The Forgotten Future

Can you come up here for a little while? We have a patient who needs a one-to-one and there's no one else to do it."

Had it been an adult patient, I probably would have refused. But it was a kid.

I had never met Lavonne, but Jackie gave me a quick report while we walked to her room. "She came in this afternoon and was okay at first. When I went in to do her vitals about half an hour ago, though, she was curled up in a little ball on her bed just crying and staring. She got really freaked out when I walked over to her. Dr. Evans is in with her now."

We walked into the room where Lavonne was still curled up on her bed. Knees to her chest, arms bent and pulled in tight, fists clinched. Dr. Evans sat in a chair by the bed and stood as we entered. Ever the gentleman, he spoke to Lavonne. "Lavonne, this is Debbi. She's a good nurse who's going to stay with you for a while. She's very nice and easy to talk to. I'm going to leave for a few minutes, but if you need me, just let Debbi know."

Evans and I nodded to each other as I took his seat, and he followed Jackie out the door. I spoke quietly. "Hi Lavonne, how are you doing?"

No response.

"I heard you just got here this afternoon. Is that right? I usually work here on the adolescent unit, but today they sent me to work with the adults." I smiled at her, even though she wasn't looking. "I like working with you guys better."

I continued talking as I watched Lavonne for some movement, some utterance, *something,* that might give us a clue as to what was going on with her. Twenty minutes or so later, I noticed her eyes darting rapidly around the room. She still hadn't moved. Just her eyes. And she looked scared. Real scared. Then she tucked her head down close to her chest. Her eyes still followed something around the room that I couldn't see.

Suddenly, she stuck both hands between her legs and grabbed her crotch. She let out a blood-curdling scream and began to writhe on the bed. I watched as she flailed about, crying and fighting back at the demons tormenting her. Then, just as quickly, she was still. And quiet.

I recognized what had transpired, and I asked softly, "Is there anything I can do, Lavonne?"

She shook her head almost imperceptibly. "No," she whispered, "he's gone."

A few moments later I filled Jackie in on what had happened, and she sat with Lavonne while I joined Dr. Evans in the nurses' office. I told him about Lavonne's episode, and he nodded. "I suspected that she had been abused." He leaned back in the chair. "We don't want to pressure her, but we need to try to find out who did this to her. My hunch, and it's only a hunch, is that it was her older brother." He sat up straight. "Can you stay with her for the rest of the shift?"

After Jackie joined me in the hall, she told me "it" had happened again. Jackie had tears in her eyes, and she was shaking. "Oh, my god, Debbi! I've never seen anyone like that before ... it was like, like ... like she was being tortured right in front of me!"

I thought of Billy from so many years before and knew how she felt. Like all her innocence was gone forever. Lord Byron's "heavenly ignorance" was no more. I touched her cheek and breathed, "I know. I know."

*　　*　　*　　*

Pervasive throughout all societies and cultures, mental illness impacts families, friends, employers, schools, and our health and judicial systems. National Institute of Mental Health (NIMH) researchers have found that, unlike most disabling physical diseases, mental illness begins early in life. Half of all lifetime cases of mental illness begin by age fourteen, and three-quarters begin by age twenty-four. Understanding this, we are beginning to understand that mental disorders are really the chronic diseases of the young

Despite today's effective treatments—psychotherapy and medication—there are often long delays—years or sometimes even decades—between the onset of symptoms and the time when people actually seek and receive treatment. The NIMH study reveals that an untreated mental disorder can lead to a more severe, more diffi-

The Forgotten Future

cult-to-treat, mental illness and to the development of co-occurring mental illnesses at a later time. Nearly half (45 percent) of those with any mental disorder meet the criteria for two or more disorders.

We need to acknowledge the prevalence of mental illness in our young people and the toll taken by such illnesses, we must make it a priority to properly diagnose and effectively treat our children before it is too late, and we must look beyond the palliative fixes offered by some to long-term treatment solutions that will yield achieving, creative, fulfilled, contented and productive members of society.

Until we do, there will continue to be—every day—kids whose troubled minds will wreak havoc on themselves and on others. For family members and mental health professionals alike, there will always be a new story to hear and a shocking new detail to learn. There will always someone who mental health professionals want to help—someone we want to help with every fiber of our being and with whatever resources or talents we can muster. There will be kids like

the kid who stabbed his father in the face because his father had turned off the video game to watch the news,

the kid who had committed two rapes and numerous molestations by the time he was twelve,

the kid who repeatedly "flashed" any female in sight,

the kid who drank so much that she suffered a cardiac arrest, yet within six weeks was back swigging at parties,

the kid who injected his cat with cocaine, and the one who set the neighbor's dog on fire,

the kids who stole cars, who cut themselves for attention, and the ones who slip through the cracks, and

the kids who abuse and are themselves abused.

In never-ending supply.

Chapter 10
Changes

The patients' telephone in the community room rang harshly, but there were no children to answer it. Moments before, they had all been unceremoniously whisked away to the safety of the hospital school. The phone rang and rang—perhaps 20 rings—and then it dawned on me: *She doesn't know. She doesn't know her son is dead. She expects him to answer the phone.*

I heard someone in the office say, "That's his mother. Andrew's mother. She was supposed to call him this morning."

The ringing stopped.

I stood outside the office door, listening to the discussion inside: *Well, somebody has to talk to her; you know she's going to call back. What do we want to say? Who's going to talk to her?*

The phone rang again.

I waited impatiently for a few rings and then leaned into the office and asked if anyone was going to answer the phone. I spoke in a tone that was intentionally sharper than my usual style, more demanding, but I was disturbed by their delay in answering the phone. I realized that talking to Lucinda McClain was going to be difficult, but she deserved to know what had happened. As the evening coordinator, I didn't have the authority to speak to her about something like the untimely death of her son, and I didn't want to answer the phone and be put into the position of having to evade her questions.

Apparently, there was still no agreement about who was going to speak with Ms. McClain because I continued to hear hurried whispers discussing who and what and how. The hospital administrators, including Michael Suchopar, Elmcrest's vice president of operations, seemed to be waiting for someone to make some sort of decision. The ringing continued.

I remained at the office door, glaring and wondering when someone would stand up and speak to Andrew's mother. Finally, Brian Fay, the children's unit's program director, came into the community room to answer the call.

Andrew's mother wanted to speak to him. She also wanted to know why it took so long to answer the phone. Their conversation was brief. Brian explained that there was a problem and Andrew was not on the unit. He told her to go to Middlesex Hospital where they would give her more information.

*   *   *   *

My own phone at home had rung a few minutes after nine that Sunday morning. I ignored it.

It was my day off, and I was exhausted. There was a late-season New England blizzard blowing, and while working full-time on a children's unit was a job I loved, it was also tiring, and my weekends were a time to regroup. With the outside temperature hovering at an unseasonable eight degrees, my bed and my comforter were quite warm and comfortable, thank you very much.

My sleepy teenage son dragged himself into my room and told me it was Donna from the hospital calling. I groaned.

I lifted my head from the pillow. "I'm not working today; I'm too tired. Tell her I'm sleeping and I'll call her back later."

Donna was the weekend nursing supervisor, and I knew her call meant she wanted me to come in to work. No, I reassured myself, there's no way I'm working today. I pulled the comforter tight under my chin and snuggled deeper into the warmth as Jon returned to the phone in his room.

The Forgotten Future

Almost two years previously, I had accepted the position of Evening Coordinator at Elmcrest Psychiatric Institute in Portland, Connecticut, and had begun working on a children's unit with children between the ages of three and twelve. Many of these children had problems similar to those of the teens with whom I had previously worked, but I hoped the younger kids would offer a fresh perspective on mental illness in young people. I also hoped that I would find that earlier intervention would provide a measure of effectiveness that often eluded us with the teens.

"Uh, mom ..." Jon was at my door again. "She sounds really mad. She said to tell you to get out of bed, that she really needs to talk to you right now."

I stumbled to the phone and mumbled a greeting of sorts.

"Debbi? We've got some problems here, and we need you to come in." Donna sounded pressured.

I closed my eyes. "Uh, do you really need me, Donna? I'm beat, and I need a break."

"Andrew McClain went into cardiac arrest during a restraint this morning—the EMTs are getting him ready for transport to Middlesex Hospital now." She paused. "We really need you here. Things are a mess."

Andrew was an eleven-year-old who had been admitted during the early morning hours the previous Thursday and who was on the unit when I worked Thursday and Friday evenings. Having met him only twice, I knew little about him. He was easy to picture, though, mostly due to his prosthetic eye, the result of an early-childhood injury that had not received proper medical attention.

His story was akin to many that I had encountered over the years—troubled family life, serial foster homes, problem behavior. Born to a thirteen-year-old mother, he was the product of a family whose social services needs had been neglected for generations. In addition to that brief history, we had also been told that Andrew had recently threatened to kill his foster brother and had reportedly placed cleaning chemicals on the younger child's toothbrush several times over a three-week period.

I told Donna that I would be there as soon as I could and quickly got dressed. Driving the twenty-plus miles to the hospital, I had time to mull over what Donna had told me. I tried to imagine the scene. With emergency response personnel arriving at the hospital, I was sure there was real excitement in the air. After all, they were just kids.

At the same time, I knew there were twenty-six children of varying ages on the unit, and something like this was sure to have frightened them. It was hard to imagine anything really serious happening on the children's unit, however, and I even had a passing notion that there might have been a mistake or overreaction and Andrew would be back on the unit by the time I arrived. Oh well, I thought, I'm awake now, and it'll be a relaxing day with the kids once Andrew comes back from the emergency room. Maybe we would go out and play in the fresh snow.

When I arrived at Elmcrest, I found the unit nurses' office packed with administrative personnel, staff from other units, and our unit's staff from other shifts who had been called in to help deal with the crisis. Everyone looked stunned; silence filled the office. People clung to each other and rocked back and forth, seeking strength, seeking comfort.

Andrew had been pronounced dead at 10:17.

The unimaginable had happened.

Dead. I turned the word over in my mind, trying to make some sense of it, some association between the lively, *alive,* kids with whom I worked and what I had just been told had happened. It didn't connect.

Karen Slonus, the part-time registered nurse in charge of the unit that morning, and the two mental health techs involved in the restraint, Jen Bryant and Spero Parasco, were in the back corner of the office.

Jen sat cross-legged on the floor, fists clenched. She rocked back and forth, sobbing and moaning, like a wounded being. At times, it was almost as if she were not even present as she stared into space, seemingly trying to make sense of everything.

Of something.

Of anything.

Spero sat alone, head down, hands visibly shaking. He looked dazed, as if he wasn't quite sure what had happened. Then, suddenly, he looked into my eyes and cried out, "We killed him!" I understood what he meant; there was no doubt in my mind. He was in pain and was so confused over the outcome of an action that he had taken to protect a patient that the irrational statement was all he could think of to say.

My eyes welled. There was nothing that I could do or say to comfort any of them. Nothing at all. My heart broke as I realized that there was more than one victim in this horrible scene unfolding before me.

Lost in my own thoughts, unable to find words of solace for my co-workers, I began to think and wonder what I might have felt had I been directly involved in Andrew's death instead of Jen or Karen or Spero. Would I have blamed myself, would I have second-guessed my actions with Andrew? Would I have responded differently in the emergency?

What could have gone wrong? What had happened to cause Andrew's death?

I heard someone ask, "Are all the kids off the unit? The police want to come in." I turned and answered to no one in particular, "Yeah. They're at the gym and then they'll be up at the school."

Because I had not been directly involved in the morning's tragedy and because I knew that the remaining children still had to be cared for, I went to prepare the mid-morning med pass. As I watched from the relative sanctuary of the med room, I saw the Portland Police and the Connecticut State Police Eastern District Major Crime Squad seal the entrance to the timeout room with yellow "crime scene" tape. It was disconcerting to think of any part of the unit as a crime scene when the unit, these rooms, had been a place where previously I had been just as comfortable as in my own home. Even on those evenings when the unit was chaotic, and one or more kids was out of control—kicking or spitting or biting or hitting or throwing furniture—I knew the routine and the plan and had a pretty good picture of the outcome.

I finished pouring the meds and walked to the office where Andrew's chart and medication sheet were being meticulously studied by the hospital's administrators. Medical data, including Andrew's admission history, physical, and lab work, were reviewed and then photocopied for closer inspection later. They were searching for something that might have been missed at the time of Andrew's admission that could have contributed to his untimely death and, at the same time, copying the chart to review later, after the police took the hardcopy paper chart. I watched from outside the door.

Then the phone rang. Lucinda McClain was trying to reach her son.

*   *   *   *

Visiting hours on Sundays were from 1:00 to 2:00 in the afternoon. In order to prevent the children's visitors from inadvertently going to the unit where the police investigation was in progress, this day all visitors were met in the main reception area and escorted to the hospital school.

Most of the children didn't have visitors. Ever. Many of the children hospitalized at Elmcrest were no longer connected to, or involved with, their biological families, and many times the children were in-between foster homes. Even in those cases in which there are interested family members, they often have no transportation to the hospital. On that Sunday, there were three, maybe four, visitors.

One of the younger boys was visited by both parents, and he excitedly told them, "Andrew got sick and had to go to the hospital this morning." His mother patiently explained that *this is the hospital* and *this* is where Andrew is.

As they talked, I listened carefully. I don't believe she knew who Andrew was; she just assumed that he was another child on the unit. Her son kept trying to make her understand, saying, "But, but, but ..." and "No! *Another* hospital!", but she never understood what he was trying to tell her. I sat quietly with one of the mental health techs, watching the kids, hoping the child's mother wouldn't come over and ask me any questions. She didn't, and I was relieved, for I had no answers.

I relaxed a little after visiting hours were over. I looked at my watch and realized it was almost 3:00. The office remained hectic, with people coming and going, and the evening staff started to arrive. Those who hadn't already heard about Andrew were told what had happened. Everyone was shocked, but quickly asked where they were needed most, and I sent them up to the school to relieve the exhausted day staff.

Around 4:00, the unit's clinical staff arrived to be available when we told the kids about Andrew's death. We had decided that it was important that they learn about Andrew directly from us, and I hoped we could provide an appropriate explanation.

The children filed in from the school and were directed straight to the burgundy rubber couches in the center of our community room. This is where we ordinarily held group meetings and where the children gathered before leaving the building for school or gym. They didn't seem to notice the unusual number of staff people standing around, lining the walls: nurses, mental health techs and clinicians who were not scheduled to work weekends. The children knew everyone's schedule—days and times—and if a staff person was in on the "wrong" day or time, the child usually called it to their attention immediately.

This day they made no comment.

Maybe they intuitively knew why.

Members of the staff explained that Andrew had gone to the other hospital that morning because he had stopped breathing. His heart had stopped beating, and the doctors had worked very, very hard to get it started again, but there was nothing they could do, and he had died. There were a couple of gasps from the group, and some of the children started to cry. Softly.

Some of our kids had intimate knowledge of death—it's not unusual these days for children to have a relative, even a parent, who has died from drugs, violence, or AIDS or other diseases. Some of the kids, however, were so young that their concept of death was unclear. We talked briefly about the meaning of death and reassured the kids that they were safe. The clinicians, nurses and mental health techs made it clear that they were available to any child who needed consoling or just wanted to talk.

One of the children quietly raised his hand. When called upon, he gently asked if we could have a moment of silence for Andrew.

Deborah Clark Ebel, R.N.

In that room of mourning, the silence was deafening.

Later that night, safe at home, I watched the 11:00 news. Andrew's death was the lead story. The reality of what had happened overwhelmed me, and I was consumed by feelings I had suppressed all day—sadness, despair, fear, horror, confusion. I began sobbing the first tears of many that would flow for months. I didn't sleep that night.

* * * *

The next day, Monday, the entire unit staff, including the hospital school teachers, were telephoned and told of a mandatory 1:30 meeting. The preliminary autopsy report was to be released at 2:00.

Nurses, mental health techs, clinicians, and school teachers gathered around a table in the conference room. The somber formal portraits of the founder and past directors of the hospital stared down at us as Brian Fay reviewed the previous day's events and went into more detail for those who had not been present.

All around, there were expressions of support for the staff involved in the restraint. But while we all were deeply concerned for the three staff members, our supportive utterances were as much about our own fears as they were about our co-workers' well-being.

Brian cleared his throat as he listened to us talk, and then he warned us that the autopsy results might not turn out the way we hoped. I knew then, in my heart, that he already knew the results. He could not, and would not, tell us until the report was officially released. But he knew.

Michael Suchopar entered promptly at 2:00 and quietly slipped into a chair near the end of the table. He sighed deeply and looked exhausted. He told us that the preliminary autopsy report had been released, and it indicated that Andrew had died of traumatic asphyxiation.

Suffocation.

It was the outcome we had feared most, and it stirred all our innermost doubts and fears. Most of us had hoped that Andrew had

~ 224 ~

died from some pre-existing medical condition and not through anything the staff had done, but a few of us had discussed the possibility that he might have died from suffocation due to the type of restraint that had been used. While we were devastated by the death of a child in our care, to think that an action done by any one of us might have contributed to his death in any way was overwhelming. Most frightening of all was the fact that we had all participated in countless restraints just like the one that killed Andrew.

The heartbreak in the room was palpable. Some sat silently; some sobbed openly. Sadness saturated us. For Andrew, his mother and ourselves. For all the children.

Following a brief discussion, Suchopar left for a hospital-wide meeting to inform the rest of the hospital staff about the autopsy results. After he left, members of the children's unit staff stood silently, embracing, seeking some strength, some solace, from one another. Some prayed. Then, after there was nothing left to say, we slowly returned to the unit where twenty-five children still very much needed us.

*　　*　　*　　*

The single memorable exchange that I had with Andrew was when I had given him his medications on Thursday evening. He took nortriptyline, an antidepressant, and risperidone, a powerful antipsychotic used to help control his violent behavior. He put the pills into his mouth and gave me a steady, almost challenging, look.

"Did you swallow them? Or are you messing with me?" I asked.

Patients not infrequently "cheek" their meds and spit them out when they think the nurse is not looking. They don't like the side effects, which can range from dry mouth to lethargy to disorientation to serious weight gain.

Andrew held his gaze, but he didn't answer. He opened his mouth and moved his tongue from side to side to show me that he had swallowed. Then he turned sideways to watch me with his good eye.

My gut feeling was that he hadn't actually swallowed the pills, so I told him that I wanted him to stay with me at the med room. Eventually the pills would melt, and he would have to swallow. I started my usual explanation about meds and the reasons and importance of taking them, but Andrew wasn't listening.

I wasn't surprised when I later read Andrew's autopsy report and noted the "zero" blood level of risperidone, the antipsychotic. Antipsychotics in children are used to treat, among other things, self-injurious behavior and uncontrollable aggression. The day he died, Andrew went to the timeout room and was restrained after threatening another boy and refusing to follow the mental health tech's directions.

The level of "zero" risperidone meant that Andrew had been cheeking his meds, and, as a result, he was not receiving any benefit from the drug intended to help him keep his frequently violent behavior under control. He was at the mercy of his mental illness.

*   *   *   *

The use of seclusion and restraint has long been debated in the psychiatric community. Most clinicians agree that when a patient loses control to the extent that he or she is at imminent risk of physical harm to self or others, staff may legitimately restrain the patient *as an emergency measure.* There is far less agreement regarding the use of restraint and seclusion in other situations, however.

Physical restraint and seclusion in any situation can be dangerous because the act of restraining a patient can involve a physical struggle and some sort of pressure on the patient's chest. Known causes of death in which restraint or seclusion have been a factor include asphyxia, cardiac complications, drug overdoses or interactions, blunt trauma, strangulation or choking, and aspiration. Injuries suffered by patients who have been restrained range from having teeth knocked out to bruises and lacerations to fractured ribs and other broken bones.

The frequent use of per-diem, float, or agency staff to compensate for inadequate numbers of full-time permanent staff leaves a void to be filled by workers who are unfamiliar with individual patients' temperaments, behaviors, needs, and comorbid (co-existing) medical conditions. Not knowing the unit population or unit standards frequently leads these staff persons to over-enforce consequences or misinterpret patient behavior and institute unnecessary seclusion or restraint. In Andrew McClain's case, all of the staff on the unit the morning that he died were either part-time, per-diem, or float staff. Consequently, they were unfamiliar with Andrew's background and behavioral triggers, and Andrew was restrained unnecessarily.

I would be remiss if I failed to here make note that workers in the mental health care system are also often injured, at times seriously. Repeated studies show that most staff injuries in mental health facilities are sustained when staff are trying to control patient violence and during restraint or seclusion incidents.

*   *   *   *

In the months following Andrew McClain's death, a team of reporters from The Hartford Courant, the newspaper covering the region in which Elmcrest is located, compiled a database of 142 restraint-related patient deaths which had occurred in psychiatric hospitals, psychiatric wards of general hospitals, group homes, and similar facilities during the previous ten years. The exact number of deaths that actually occurred due to restraint or seclusion is unknown because, at that time, New York was the only state which mandated reporting of such deaths.

As part of its investigation, The Hartford Courant engaged the services of research statistician Roberta J. Glass of the Harvard Center for Risk Analysis at the Harvard School of Public Health. Using data from the state of New York and the United States Department of Health and Human Services, along with earlier studies on the use of restraints, Ms. Glass projected that the annual number of restraint-related deaths could be as high as 150 and further stated her belief that deaths and injuries from seclusion and restraints are significantly underreported. Her estimates include all ages; however, a disproportionate number of restraint-related deaths occur in children.

Deborah Clark Ebel, R.N.

The Hartford Courant series sparked a series of high-profile congressional hearings that set out to examine the use of seclusion and restraint as a form of behavior management in mental health facilities. During these hearings, deaths, injuries, and abuses that had occurred during or following seclusion or restraint were brought to light, and for the first time, the public was made aware of the far-reaching use of these measures and the fact that deaths from such measures were a not-uncommon outcome of such measures.

"Unfortunately, these are not isolated incidents. They are but a few of scores of cases in which mental health patients—a disproportionate number of them children—died barbaric deaths more suited to medieval torture chambers than to late 20th century America. They died because of the improper use of seclusion and physical or chemical restraints. They died at the hands of the very people who were supposed to protect them."
---Senator Joseph Lieberman, Senator Christopher Dodd, and Representative Rosa DeLauro, July 16, 1999

Following these hearings, and with prompting from national mental health advocacy groups, the federal government stepped in to improve the situation. In July, 1999, the Centers for Medicare and Medicaid Services (CMS) issued interim rules on the use of restraints for Medicare- and Medicaid-funded hospitals. These directives focused on practices that must be taken into consideration when restraining a patient.

The federal Children's Health Act of 2000 was a step toward reform when it established the first national standards for the use of restraints and seclusion in psychiatric facilities. Also, for the first time, facilities receiving federal funds were required to notify appropriate state licensing or regulatory agencies of any death occurring at their facility within 24 hours.

In late 2006, more than eight-and-a-half years after Andrew McClain's death, the federal government issued its final rules governing the use of restraints and seclusion on patients in Medicare- and Medicaid-funded hospitals. These new rules and regulations include time limits on seclusion and physical restraints, as well as time periods during which a patient held in restraints must be evaluated face-to-face by a physician. Facilities are now required to document the reason for the seclusion or restraint, as well as what attempts at less-restrictive methods were used and how the patient responded to those interventions.

The rules impacting Medicare- and Medicaid-funded hospitals do not apply to other types of mental health facilites, but many of these other facilities have put forth seclusion and restraint policies of their own. These facility-initiated protocols, however, are merely guidelines, without any outside monitoring or consequences for noncompliance, and how much effect these policies will ultimately have on actual practice remains to be seen.

Unfortunately, while the situation in hospitals appears to have improved under government pressure, overly-aggressive restraints continue in many other types of facilities—day treatment centers, residential treatment centers, boot camps, treatment academies, and others—and have continued to result in deaths.

In May, 2006, seven-year-old Angellika Arndt died at Rice Lake Day Treatment Center in Wisconsin after being placed in a "control hold" as a consequence for misbehaving. During the hour she was kept in a dangerous face-down prone restraint, she cried for help, saying she could not breathe. She vomited, urinated, and defecated on herself. The medical examiner ruled Angellika's death a homicide due to "complications from chest compression asphyxiation".

In January, 2007, seventeen-year-old Isaiah Simmons died after being restrained at Bowling Brook Preparatory School, a private residential school for court-committed adolescent males in Maryland. Isaiah's death has raised serious questions about state laws governing privately run facilities, the training required of their staff, and the way the state monitors and regulates such programs.

In June, 2007, seventeen-year-old Omega Leach died after two staff members at the Chad Youth Enhancement Center in Tennessee restrained him for unruly behavior. He had been in at least eight treatment centers and mental hospitals over a period of xix years. State regulators concluded that a Chad staffer had provoked a confrontation that led to Leach's death.

*   *   *   *

The death of Andrew McClain had an unexpectedly profound effect on me, and several months after his death, I decided to take some time to reevaluate the direction my life and career were taking. I knew that before I could continue working in the mental health field, I had to really examine society's relationship to, and treatment, of children. I had to come to an understanding in my own mind of what I believed our nation's responsibility regarding the care and safety of our children to be, and I had to look at who is responsible for ensuring that all children receive care that is appropriate to their needs. Falling back on my knowledge of, and experience in, psychiatric facilities, I had to look squarely at the treatment provided to a large number of young people today and try to call our nation's attention to the fact that not only are many millions of our children suffering from mental illnesses, but the system itself is seriously troubled.

The conditions and situations leading to the placement of so many of our children in psychiatric hospitals and residential treatment facilities and the like are far more commonplace than the public has acknowledged or would like to believe. It hurts to have an awareness of such things, so, for the most part, society wears blinders when it comes to the atrocities perpetrated on countless children. We become indignant over isolated media reports of abuse, yet thousands of children and teenagers contend with maltreatment every day of their lives. It's not something that's easy to think about, so we don't.

I wondered whether or not I could ever return to working with children.

After leaving Elmcrest, I cried off and on for the first week, questioning my decision to leave and sorrowing for Andrew. Physically and emotionally drained, my initial focus was my failure to "hang in there". I couldn't see the good I had accomplished over the years, nor accept that it was time stand back and take a second look at where I was going.

The Forgotten Future

My head ached, my stomach churned. I slept a lot, sometimes waking to find my pillow soaked with tears. I went through a horrible array of emotions leading up to, and following, my decision: sadness, fear, anger, embarrassment. Gradually, I came to see the situation as it really was. I had done a difficult job for many years and had given it my best. Now I needed a change.

Still, it was hard to imagine a professional life that didn't include working with kids.

One evening, months after leaving Elmcrest, my son and I entered a local supermarket. I heard someone shout, "Hey!" but paid no attention.

"Hey!" again. More urgent. "Don't you work at Elmcrest?"

I suddenly felt warm and flush as I turned to face my accuser. "I used to …" Several teenage boys stood about fifteen feet away, and I searched faces.

"Here! Over here!" A boy, about fourteen, stood waving his hands wildly. Our eyes met, and he grinned. I recognized him immediately and smiled. He took a couple of hesitant steps forward and then broke into a run until we were hugging. He hugged me tight, and I held on like I hadn't done in months. It felt good. My eyes stung.

"How are you?" I pulled away and looked at someone so familiar, yet from another time and place. "Your family?"

"Good. I'm good." He turned toward one of his friends and yelled, "Hey, dude! Make him get off my bike!" He shifted from foot to foot and asked, "What do you mean you *used* to work at Elmcrest? Don't you work there anymore?"

"No …"

He cut in, "How come?"

My mind raced with the answer to his question and the answer *was because I didn't think what was happening there was therapeutic or helping you or good enough for you. I thought the system was ineffective and you guys deserve better. Because I simply couldn't stand the pain anymore.* That was my answer, but I couldn't say that, so I simply said, "I just decided to take a long vacation."

He cocked his head to the side and narrowed his eyes. "Man,

that's too bad. You were good, too." He took a step backward. "I gotta go. He's bein' a jerk with my bike."

A high-five, and he was gone.

I was shaking. My throat was tight and my eyes were damp. I remembered he had no family, at least no real family he could count on. The last time I saw him, his dad was on a binge and his mom didn't want him back at home. There was no foster home available; two had already fallen through.

I realized then how very much I missed the kids. I had blocked it out for months and tried to pretend it didn't matter, but it did. I remembered now why I had become a nurse in the first place, why I had done the job I did for as long as I had.

I could never forget them.

My heart ached.

Appendix A
What to do if Your Teen is troubled

Given all that you've just read about the current state of mental health care in America, you may be wondering what to do if your own child has an emotional or behavioral problem or if you fear your child may have a mental illness. You may be worried and have many questions, but how do you know for certain that your child's situation is one that requires professional help? How should you handle behavior that seems so out of control? How do you decide what to do and where to go? What is the best course of treatment? What about medication? Will it help, or is it dangerous? And what about hospitalization? Does it ever help in any way?

You see changes in your child's emotions or behavior—sometimes bizarre or frightening ones—and you wonder whether those changes are normal variables in personality and behavior or whether they signal a serious problem. You have so many questions and so many things to think about, and you worry whether any decisions you make will be the right ones. Everyone offers advice—from relatives and friends to advice columnists in magazines or on television shows.

The information in this chapter will provide you with guidance in making some important decisions and in locating resources. You will learn signs that may indicate that your child has a problem and learn when to contact a professional. You will learn whom to approach and what questions to ask.

Please be aware, however, that none of this information is intended for diagnosis. ***Appropriate diagnosis can only be done by a qualified physician or other mental health professional,*** and you should seek professional assistance if you believe your young person has a problem. I can't stress this strongly enough. Seek help, *professional* help, if your child's emotions or behaviors seem unusual. A book or online assistance can only provide general information and direction—you must take action on your own.

This is the time to work on good communication with your teen. When you approach your child about changes in his behavior or other changes that you are concerned about, he may not want to talk about it. Your child may become angry and accuse you of meddling in his business. You must try to move beyond this. Do not become accusatory or defensive.

Begin the conversation by reminding him that you love him and that you are there for him, no matter what. Let him know that he can trust you, that he has not done anything that cannot be worked out, and that you want to know what's on his mind so you can help him.

If you're concerned about your teenager, trust your instincts. You know your child best. Parents are usually the first ones to notice that their child has a problem. You know his or her usual mood and reactions to situations. You know his or her level of functioning, and if something seems not quite as it should, you should check it out. It's far better to be proactive and address situations early on than to have to play catch-up with your child's well-being. Stay on top of things.

Today's health care system can be hard to maneuver. The mental health care system, in particular, can be complicated and difficult to understand. In a time of crisis, it can be frightening and intimidating, but the system *can* be navigated with a little information and patience.

Immediately discard any prejudices and fears you may hold about mental illness and resolve to do what is best for your child. Mental health services and treatment modalities are evolving every day. As in any field, the qualifications and abilities of those with whom you and your child will be working vary considerably from person to person. In some cases, medication may be beneficial; in others, psychotherapy alone may do the trick. In still other cases, hospitalization may be necessary to deal with the crisis.

While there is no tidy checklist of signs to determine whether or not your teen has a mental health issue, you should be aware that the following should be evaluated.

- Thinking or talking about suicide
- Threats of self-harm or harm to others
- Trouble coping with problems and daily activities
- Strange or grandiose ideas
- Expressions of worthlessness or guilt
- Excessive anxiety
- Prolonged sadness or depression or apathy
- Marked changes in eating or sleeping patterns; excessive sleeping or sleeping too little; lethargy
- Little interest in activities once enjoyed
- Notable personality change
- Extreme highs and lows
- Abuse of alcohol and/or drugs
- Excessive anger, hostility, or violent behavior
- Abuse of animals
- Marked change in school performance
- Frequent physical complaints, such as headaches or digestive problems
- Persistent nightmares
- Threatening to run away or running away

A teenager displaying one or more of these warning signs should be seen and evaluated by a psychiatrist or other physician as quickly as possible. This evaluation may take place in the practitioner's office or in your local hospital's emergency room. Before discussing what you should expect from such an evaluation, however, below are some suggestions about where to find a mental health professional.

Where to Find Help

If you need help right away and your child is willing to safely accompany you, seek assistance at a nearby hospital emergency room. If you believe your child poses an immediate danger to himself or to anyone else, and you think—even remotely—that you might have trouble transporting him to the emergency room yourself, *immediately dial 911*. Do not concern yourself with what the neighbors might think. This is an emergency and must be handled as such.

If your child is having difficulties that do not pose an immediate crisis, but you are still concerned about his recent behavior or emotional state, your first contact might be your child's pediatrician or family physician—your primary care physician (PCP). Call the doctor's office and tell the receptionist that your child needs to be seen as quickly as possible, preferably the same or next day. When the appointment time is set, make sure that you keep the appointment. If your child's other parent is available, he or she should accompany you.

In addition to asking about your child's recent behavior, your PCP will most likely want to perform a thorough physical examination of your child and do appropriate laboratory tests to determine whether any medical illness might be contributing to your child's symptoms.

You may find that your child's PCP wants to be the sole care provider for your child. While your PCP can certainly prescribe medication such as antidepressants or ADHD medications for your child, be aware that PCPs are not trained in psychiatry or psychology and that you will have to go elsewhere for the talk-therapy component of your child's treatment. Sometimes a PCP may provide brief counseling, but, as you know, your PCP's time is limited, and he or she does not have the "fifty-minute hour" that mental health professionals normally provide.

Additionally, there is evidence that mental disorders often go undiagnosed, untreated, or undertreated when PCPs are the sole caregivers for mental health issues, and without proper intervention, child and adolescent disorders frequently continue into adulthood and can seriously impair your child's chances of developing into a competent, responsible adult.

If you believe that your child has a serious mental health problem and/or you believe that your child has not improved sufficiently under the PCP's care, it is important to seek assistance from someone more knowledgeable and experienced in mental health issues, i.e., a psychiatrist or other mental health professional. Please do not sacrifice you child's future in order to avoid hurting the feelings of your child's PCP. Trust that your PCP will ultimately want what's best for your child.

If your child does not have a regular physician, ask your child's school counselor or your clergyperson for a referral to a professional with expertise in adolescent mental health. One thing to be aware of here is that while clergy can be helpful in crises of a spiritual nature, mental health problems require specialized assistance. Most clergy have limited exposure to, or education in, what is required to adequately and properly address mental health problems, and I recommend that you consult a mental health professional. Your church or synagogue may be able to put you in touch with a pastoral counseling program if a spiritual component is important to you, and these centers are usually staffed by mental health professionals.

Another possibility when seeking a referral is to ask family members or friends for their recommendations, especially if their adolescent has had a good experience with psychotherapy. A referral from family or friends whose opinion you trust can be invaluable, but do not accept a diagnosis from friends or family just because they tell you that their "son/daughter had the same problem … acted the same way and the doctor said he/she has …'' Behaviors have many causes, and similarities between different illnesses may come into play. Only a professional can adequately and appropriately provide diagnosis.

Additionally, taking medication that is not specifically prescribed for a patient is extremely dangerous. Do not accept medications—not even over-the-counter medications—from friends or family members, even if they insist that the medication helped in a situation similar to your child's. Psychotropic medications work on the brain, and you do not want to give your child such medication unless it is ordered and monitored by a physician.

The division of adolescent psychiatry or department of psychology in any medical school or university may provide a referral to a competent professional. Medical and psychiatric societies can tell you where psychiatrists attended medical school, where they did their residencies, and whether they are certified by the American Board of Psychiatry and Neurology. Board certification is desirable. You should feel free to specify age, sex, race, ethnicity, or religious background of the doctor if that is important to you.

Call or visit your community mental health center, mental health association, or a support group such as the local chapter of the Federation of Families for Children's Mental Health (FFCMH) or the National Alliance on Mental Illness (NAMI). They may have a list of mental health professionals in your area who are accepting new patients. National contact information for some of these organizations is listed in Appendix B, and you can also find information at libraries and on the Internet.

Your employer may offer an Employee Assistance Program (EAP) that may be able to steer you in the right direction. An EAP is a benefit from your employer, and many provide assistance to employees and their families for substance abuse, stress-related illnesses, depression, and other mental health issues. Visits are generally free, but there are usually a limited number of visits allowed. Although engaged by your employer, the EAP is bound by confidentially laws to keep your business private and your employer will not be notified that you have sought help from the EAP nor given information about issues discussed in your sessions.

Once your child's medical doctor or other source has given you suggestions and if you're not facing an emergency situation, select two or three possible psychiatrists and phone for information about appointment availability, location, and cost of the first visit. Weigh all your options, choose a provider, and schedule an appointment. Don't be shy about stressing to your contact the immediacy of your need for a quick appointment.

Who's Who and What do All the Letters Mean?

A child and adolescent psychiatrist is a fully-trained and licensed medical doctor (M.D.) or osteopathic physician (D.O.) who has been specially trained in psychiatry and who has at least two additional years of advanced training dealing with children, adolescents, and families beyond medical school and general psychiatric training. Choose a psychiatrist who is board certified in child and adolescent psychiatry by the American Board of Psychiatry and Neurology. Psychiatrists—because they are licensed physicians—are the only mental health professionals who can prescribe and monitor medications to help restore imbalances in body chemistry that many believe are related to mental illness.

Some psychologists hold masters' degrees (M.S.) and others have doctoral degrees (Ph.D., Psy.D., or Ed.D.). Psychologists are licensed in all states, and those with doctoral degrees are referred to as "Doctor". Be reminded, however, that psychologists are not medical doctors and cannot prescribe nor properly monitor medications. Psychologists specialize in psychotherapy—the "talk therapy" component of treatment. Psychologists work to understand and improve the patient's functioning at home, at school, at play, at work, and in society. There are different types of psychologists, including clinical psychologists (who offer counseling and psychotherapy and possibly psychological testing), educational or school psychologists (who work to identify academic strengths and weaknesses and specific learning disorders or developmental learning problems), neuropsychologists (who diagnosis mental and behavioral problems that are related to brain injuries), and still other types of psychologists who on focus on different areas.

A social worker holds either a bachelor's degree (B.A., B.S., or B.S.W.) or a master's degree (M.S. or M.S.W.). In most states, a social worker can take an examination to be licensed as a clinical social worker. While there are many different types of social workers, only a licensed clinical social worker (LCSW) with a master's degree in social work can provide clinical services as an independent practitioner. Social workers provide many different forms of treatment, and many are excellent at what they do.

A certified professional counselor (CPC) or a licensed professional counselor (LPC) holds a master's degree and state licensure or certification at the highest level of independent practice in the state where they practice. A marriage and family therapist is identified as either MFT or MFCC (marriage, family and child counselor) and holds a master's degree. These therapists provide assistance to troubled children and families and to individuals coping with troubled relationships

None of these professionals should be confused with the mental health workers in the earlier chapters of this book who may also be called mental health techs, mental health counselors, or psychiatric technicians. These employees are an important part of the safe management of any mental health unit, and these units could not operate safely without them. However, in most states these individuals are not required to have any special training or qualifications, and as of this writing, only four states require that psychiatric technicians be licensed—California, Kansas, Colorado, and Arkansas. Many mental health techs pursue further education or certification on their own, and in so doing, the care they provide to their patients is greatly enhanced.

You may occasionally come across an unqualified person calling himself a "counselor" and posing as someone who can help you. Unless your "counselor" has advanced training and experience with the evaluation and treatment of children, adolescents, and families, steer clear.

Seeing the Professional

At your child's first visit, the psychiatrist or other mental health professional will probably ask questions about your family's background, habits, your child's general health, and why you think your child needs treatment. (In order to avoid excessive wordiness, I will henceforth refer to the mental health professional as the "therapist" unless referring to something that only one professional, i.e., a psychiatrist, can do or provide.) The therapist will want to know when your child last had a complete physical examination and may ask your permission to consult with your child's personal physician. He will also ask about any history of mental illness on either side of your child's family.

Be honest about your child's problems as you see them and cite any specific instances of emotional or behavioral difficulties that you are able to recall. The therapist will probably see you and your child separately at the first visit in order to obtain the most information, as well as to learn about the problem as seen from both perspectives.

These days, you cannot make any assumptions about anything. Ask if the practitioner is licensed by your state, and ask their level of education. (Remember all those letters?) You should also feel free to ask questions about fees, appointment flexibility, cancellation policy, and processing of insurance forms. Ask whom you should call if you are unable to contact the doctor, especially on weekends, holidays, after hours, or in an emergency.

Good practitioners select from among many forms of psychotherapy and other treatments, depending upon your child's needs. There are psychotherapies that help patients change behaviors or thought patterns, psychotherapies that help patients explore the effect of past relationships and experiences on present behaviors, psychotherapies that treat family members together, and psychotherapies tailored to help solve other problems in specific ways. Ask what type of therapy the therapist will practice with your child and feel free to inquire about the benefits and risks of any treatment program that the psychiatrist puts before you.

When you return home after your child's initial session, ask him what he thought of the therapist. You're not asking whether or not your child thinks he needs counseling, but whether he thinks he could work with this particular professional. Think about how you both felt about the therapist and the session. What was it like to talk to someone you've never met before about personal and intimate problems? Did the therapist listen and seem to have a sense for your feelings? Is this a person you could trust? Did you like the office location and setting? Remember, your comfort and your child's comfort, both with the therapist and with the surroundings, are important considerations.

If you don't feel comfortable with the therapist and feel that this is not a "good fit", you should pay for the visit and move on to the next therapist on your list. When the chemistry does feel right, you will have taken the first step toward helping your child overcome his problems.

Deborah Clark Ebel, R.N.

Many parents are unaware of, and surprised by, the fact that information about their child's mental health and substance use is protected under confidentially laws. Parental access to records is limited, especially in the case of older adolescents. This means that you may not have access to privileged information unless your child gives permission for that access. Ask the therapist about your and your child's status with regard to confidentiality.

At your child's first appointment, if you have not already asked about the therapist's credentials, do so now. Is he a psychiatrist (i.e., a medical doctor or a doctor of osteopathy), a psychologist, a social worker, or a master's level professional counselor? Is he licensed in the state where you live?

If he is a psychiatrist, ask if he is an adolescent psychiatrist and whether he is board-certified in adolescent psychiatry.

Ask all questions in the following sections in a collegial manner, not in a confrontational or challenging manner. Assure the professional that you are not questioning his knowledge, but that you are trying to garner all the information you can about your child's condition in order to better understand the situation. Realize that you will be working in partnership with the professionals to the betterment of your child, and all the adults involved have different roles to pay.

You should ask the following:

- What is my child's diagnosis, and how did you come to make that diagnosis? *If you're not exactly sure what the doctor's words mean, ask for further explanation.*
- How often will you see my child?
- What is your hourly fee? Is this for a fifty-minute hour?
- Do you take (*whatever type of insurance you have*) insurance?
- What is your cancellation policy?
- What should I do if my child refuses to come to see you?
- Who should I call if I cannot contact you (the therapist), especially on weekends, holidays, after hours, or in an emergency?
- Do you have, or could you suggest, any reading material to

help me understand my child's illness?

How Can I Afford Care?

The fees charged by mental health professionals can range from $100 to $175 or more an hour. These fees may seem high, but you're paying for professional guidance and treatment that will impact your child's future.

Check your health insurance to see if it covers mental health treatment. All health insurance policies should include non-discriminatory coverage for psychiatric illness, although not all do. Your insurer may require a referral from your PCP before you can receive mental health services.

Many policies have limits on mental health treatment and may cover only fifty percent of the costs of a fixed number of visits per year. If your policy does not provide adequate coverage, contact your employee benefits representative or insurance agent about improving your coverage for the future. Many employers offer several health care options, and you may be able to switch to a coverage that allows for greater flexibility with psychiatric treatment, although you may have to wait for your plan's open-enrollment period to make such a change.

Even if you do not have insurance, you still have options.

If your child is already seeing a therapist, ask whether the therapist has a sliding or discounted fee schedule for cash-only patients. Such fee schedules are based on household income, and the fee goes down if you have a lower income. Unfortunately, not all therapists are able to offer a sliding fee schedule, but ask anyway. You may be able to work something out.

Your city or town may have a community mental health center that offers a reduced rate for lower-income people. The Substance Abuse and Mental Health Services Administration (SAMHSA) website in Appendix B includes a Mental Health Services Locator at which you can find mental health and substance abuse services and facilities, violence prevention services, agencies, and suicide prevention programs by city and state.

Deborah Clark Ebel, R.N.

What About Medication?

If medication is indicated and recommended, do not view this as a weakness or as a sign of failure, either of your child or your parenting. Modern psychiatric medications have allowed millions to return to their former, happier lives and have given others the opportunity to lead more satisfying and fulfilling lives for the first time.

There are many different classes of medication that are used to treat mental illness, and your child's psychiatrist will determine which meds will be most appropriate for your child's situation. The information below is provided solely to give you an idea of the wide array of medications which can be used. Be aware that there is a great deal of overlap in the use of many of these medications, and combinations of medications in the same or different class are often used for a variety of purposes. *Once again, I caution you against accepting medication of any kind from friends or relatives. Only medication that has been specifically prescribed for an individual patient should ever be taken.*

The names of medications in the following section are provided as examples of the wide variety and availability of psychiatric medications only, and are not recommended or endorsed by the author.

Many types of antidepressant medications are used in the treatment of depression, school phobia, panic attacks and other anxiety disorders, bedwetting, eating disorders, obsessive-compulsive disorder, personality disorders, and posttraumatic stress disorder (PTSD). Antidepressants are classified as selective serotonin reuptake inhibitors (SSRIs—fluoxetine {Prozac}, paroxetine {Paxil}, sertraline {Zoloft}, and many others), atypical antidepressants (duloxetine {Cymbalta}, bupropion {Wellbutron}, mirtazapine {Remeron}, and others), tricylic antidepressants (TCAs—desipramine {Norpramin}, imipramine {Tofranil}, and others), or monoamine oxidase inhibitors (MAOIs—selegiline {Emsam}, Phenelzine sulfate {Nardil}, and others), and each works in different ways.

Antipsychotic medications are used to help control psychotic symptoms such as delusions, hallucinations, or disorganized thinking, as well as to help control muscle twitches or verbal outbursts such as seen in Tourette's Syndrome. These medications are also used to treat severe anxiety and very aggressive behavior. Antipsychotic medications are classified as either first generation antipsychotic medications (chlorpromazine {Thorazine}, thioridazine hydrochloride {Mellaril}, haloperidol {Haldol}, and others) or second generation (atypical) antipsychotic medications (clozapine {Clozaril}, risperidone {Risperdal}, olanzapine {Zyprexa}, and others). In recent years, some atypical antipsychotic medications have been successful in the treatment of bipolar disorder.

Mood stabilizers and anticonvulsant medications may be used to treat severe mood swings and mood symptoms, aggressive behavior and impulse control disorders. They are also used to treat bipolar disorder. Examples of these medications include lithium, divalproex sodium (Depakoke), gabapentin (Neurontin), and others.

Benzodiazepines, such as alprazolam (Xanax), lorazepam (Ativan), diazepam (Valium), clonazepam (Klonopin), and others, as well as antihistamines, such as diphenhydramine (Benadryl) and hydroxyzine (Vistaril), are often used to treat severe anxiety. Atypical anti-anxiety medications, such as buspirone (BuSpar) have been developed and are often helpful.

Both stimulant (methylphenidate {Ritalin} and amphetamine-dextroamphetamine {Adderall}) and non-stimulant (atomoxetin {Strattera}) medications are used with children and teens diagnosed with ADHD, and there a variety of medications, such as zolpidem (Ambien) and zaleplon (Sonota), used to help on a short-term basis with sleep problems. Benadryl is commonly used on inpatient child and adolescent mental health units to help with sleep.

Some medications which are not usually thought of as psychiatric medications by the general public are actually used to treat a variety of psychiatric symptoms. For example, guanfacine (Tenex) and clonidine (Catapres), both of which are antihypertensive (high blood pressure) medications, are often used in children with conduct problems. Beta blockers, medications used to treat heart conditions and high blood pressure, are sometimes used to control "performance anxiety" when the individual must face a specific stressful situation, such as a speech, a presentation in class, or an important meeting. Propranolol (Inderal) is a beta blocker that is commonly used for such anxiety.

The single most important truth to remember about psychotropic medications is that they are powerful chemicals which alter brain chemistry. These medications can alter moods and behavior and the way that the patient perceives actions and intents, and they should be used as only one part of a comprehensive treatment plan. Continuing evaluation and monitoring by a physician is essential.

Many of these medications are prescribed for and used with children and adolescents, yet are not approved by the Food and Drug Administration (FDA) for this age group. This use is not illegal, but you should be aware that these medications have not been tested in, nor approved for, safety and efficacy in this age group. Your psychiatrist should be knowledgeable about which medications have been used successfully with different disorders, but you need to be aware that some of the medications for which you may receive samples or a written prescription have not been approved for use in children. You can check the FDA website at http://www.accessdata.fda.gov/scripts/ cder/drugsatfda/ for more information on medications.

Medications have helped many people cope with mental illness and have helped improve the quality of life for others. Some professionals, as well as consumers, however, have legitimate concerns over the use of psychotropic medications in children and adolescents. You should become as knowledgeable as possible about all aspects of your child's treatment.

If you and your child's psychiatrist decide to include medication in the treatment regime, you might want to ask some of the following questions. Include your teen in the discussion about medications, and use words that they will understand.

- What is the name of the medication? Is it known by any other name(s)? Is it available as a generic?
- How long has it been on the market?
- How much is known about this medication's safety and efficacy in children who have a condition similar to my child's?
- How will the medication help my child? What symptoms

can I expect to improve?

- How long before I see improvement?
- What are potential side effects? Are there any changes in my child that I should look for and be especially concerned about and which should be considered an emergency?
- Is this medication potentially addictive? Can it be abused?
- What is the recommended dosage? How many doses are to be given daily and how often?
- Will the dose be increased over time? What will prompt you to increase the dose? What is the maximum dose?
- Are any laboratory tests (heart tests, blood tests, etc.) needed before my child begins taking the medication? Will any tests need to be done periodically while my child is taking the medication?
- Who will monitor my child's response to medication and make changes in dosage if necessary? How often will progress be monitored and by whom?
- Are there other medications (including supplements) or foods that should be avoided while my child is taking this medication?
- How long will my child need to take this medication? How will the decision be made to stop the medication? Will my child experience negative effects over the course of discontinuing this medication?

If you still have questions or concerns or are confused about treatment options, don't hesitate ask for a second opinion.

If Your Child is Hospitalized

While you would, of course, prefer outpatient treatment, there are some situations in which you may be advised to hospitalize your child. This is a serious decision, and sometimes you must make the decision to hospitalize quickly. You're naturally concerned for your child and want the best treatment, and in an emergency situation you must do everything in your power to ensure that your child will be in an environment where he is safe.

Deborah Clark Ebel, R.N.

You may be frightened or confused when inpatient treatment is recommended. Don't hesitate to ask the following questions of your child's physician or the hospital or unit director for questions about the unit itself. You must be your son's or your daughter's strongest advocate. Most of these questions would also be appropriate if your child is going to a residential treatment center, boot camp, or other inpatient treatment facility.

- Why are you recommending inpatient treatment for my child?
- Are you the doctor who will be working with my child in the hospital?
- Are you an adolescent psychiatrist? Are you board-certified in adolescent psychiatry?
- What is my child's diagnosis, and how did you come to make that diagnosis? *If you're not exactly sure what the doctor's words mean, ask for an explanation.*
- How will inpatient hospitalization help my child?
- Are there are alternatives to hospital treatment, and, if so, how do they compare?
- How long will my child be in the hospital, and how much will it cost?
- Will I be consulted regarding any medications ordered for my child?
- What will inpatient treatment be like for my child?
- Who else will be working with my child in addition to the psychiatrist and nursing staff? *Other professionals, such as psychologists, social workers, recreation therapists, and substance abuse counselors commonly work with inpatients.*
- Are you an employee of (*the name of the hospital*) or are you an attending physician with hospital privileges?
- How many hours every day will my child actually spend in groups or individual therapy?
- Will psychological testing be done? Will I have access to the results of that testing, along with an interpretation (explanation) of the results?
- Will my child be on a unit specifically for adolescents? If

there is an adult mental health unit in the same hospital, what contact will my child have with those adult patients?

- Are males and females on separate hallways and how closely are males and females monitored during free time and after bedtime?
- Is the hospital unit accredited by the Joint Commission (JCAHO) as a treatment facility for adolescents?
- What is staffing like on the unit? How large is the unit (in other words, how many beds are on the unit?) Have you ever taken in more patients than the unit is licensed for? What is the staff-to-patient ratio, and how many registered nurses and mental health techs, each, are on each shift? *You may have to ask these questions of the hospital or unit director directly.*
- How much of the unit's staff are regular employees of the hospital *assigned to this unit*? Does the hospital use agency staff?
- How often will I receive updates on my child's status? Who will provide the updates? Do I have to call to ask for an update, and if so, who do I call?
- Who should I call with additional information that I believe is pertinent to my child's well-being?
- Is there a handbook available with information about visiting, rules, level or reward systems, anything that my child might need me to bring in, what is considered contraband, etc.?
- How are out-of-control adolescents handled? What types of restraints are used? Will I be notified by phone if my child is restrained? How soon after the restraint is initiated will I be notified? *You must understand that when a teenager is in danger of harming himself/herself or others, measures must be taken, and often decisions must be made quickly and may include restraints. You are asking these questions to ascertain that plans are in place to handle dangerous situations, not to second guess the treatment team.*

- Who provides your violence management training? Is it provided by a nationally-recognized organization? Do you have in-house trainers certified by that organization? How often is this training updated?
- What is the hospital doing to minimize the use of physical or mechanical restraints?
- Will my child be able to keep up with school work? Will my child receive work from his or her own school or will there be work substituted by the hospital? Is the unit's school accredited by the local school board?
- How can I be involved in my child's treatment, especially with regard to use of medication, discharge, and aftercare?
- How you will determine when my child is ready for discharge? How will that determination be made?
- Once my child is discharged, will be there be a plan for follow-up treatment? Who will see my child for follow-up treatment? Will I have input as to where my child is seen for this treatment?

Remember, you are not alone in having a child with a mental illness. Twenty percent of America's young people under the age of 18 suffer from mental illnesses, and between 6.4 and 9 million children have serious emotional problems. Yet, many of these children do not receive treatment.

There is hope. And by seeking out information and following the steps outlined above, you have taken the first steps toward helping your child achieve good mental health and having a rewarding future. Mental illness in adolescence is highly treatable, and by advocating for early identification and appropriate intervention, parents can make sure that their children get the help they need and ensure that their future is not forgotten.

Appendix B
Resources

The following web addresses, physical addresses, and telephone contact information may be useful in locating information to help you and your child. Agencies are listed alphabetically and hold no endorsement from the author. You may be able to find additional organizations—especially those that are disorder-specific—through Internet searches, and there are excellent books available for the layperson at libraries and booksellers. This list is not all-inclusive due to the large volume of resources.

This information is accurate as of the date of publication, and the author assumes no responsibility for changes in addresses or other contact information. Contact information changes frequently. If you are unable to access any of the web pages using the URLs provided, simply go to your browser's search feature and type in the name of the organization, service, or disorder that you are looking for. Similarly, if the phone number listed below has been changed, go to the organization's website.

American Academy of Child and Adolescent Psychiatry
3615 Wisconsin Avenue, N.W.
Washington, D.C. 20016
Phone: 202-966-7300
Website: www.aacap.org

American Association for Marriage and Family Therapy
112 South Alfred Street
Alexandria, Virginia 22314
Phone: 703-838-9808
Website: www.aamft.org

American Psychiatric Association
1000 Wilson Boulevard, Suite 1825
Arlington, Virginia 22209
Phone: (toll-free) 1-888-357-7924
Website: www.psych.org

American Psychological Association
750 First Street, N.W.
Washington, D.C. 20002
Phone: 202-336-5500
Phone: (toll-free) 1-800-374-2721
Website: www.apa.org

At Health Mental Health
Website: www.athealth.com

Judge David L. Bazelon Center for Mental Health Law
1101 15th Street, N.W., Suite 1212
Washington, D.C. 20005
Phone: 202-467-5730
Website: www.bazelon.org

Boys Town National Hotline
13940 Gutowski Road
Girls and Boys Town, Nebraska 68010
Phone: (toll-free) 1-800-448-3000
Website: www.girlsandboystown.org

The Forgotten Future

Child and Adolescent Bipolar Foundation
1000 Skokie Boulevard, Suite 570
Wilmette, Illinois 60091
Phone: 847-256-8525
Website: www.bpkids.org/site/PageServer

CHADD (Children and Adults with Attention
Deficit/Hyperactivity Disorder)
8181 Professional Place, Suite 150
Landover, Maryland 20785
Phone: 301-306-7070
Website: www.chadd.org or www.help4adhd.org

Child Help National Child Abuse Hotline
15757 North 78th Street
Scottsdale, Arizona 85260
Phone: (toll-free) 1-800-422-4453
Website: www.childhelp.org

Child Welfare League of America
440 First Street, N.W., Suite 310
Washington, D.C. 20001
Phone: 202-638-2952
Website: www.cwla.org

Covenant House Crisis Hotline
Phone: (toll-free) 1-800-999-9999
Website: www.covenanthouse.org

Depression and Bipolar Support Alliance
730 N. Franklin Street, Suite 501
Chicago, Illinois 60610
Phone: (toll-free) 1-800-826 -3632
Website: www.ndmda.org

Federation of Families for Children's Mental Health
9605 Medical Center Drive, Suite 280
Rockville, Maryland 20850
Phone: 240-403-1901
Website: www.ffcmh.org

Focus Adolescent Services
P.O. Box 4514
Salisbury, Maryland 21803
Phone: 410-341-4216
Website: www.focusas.com/index
Website: www.focusas.com/Directory.html

Internet Mental Health
Website: www.mentalhealth.com

Kids Health
Website: www.kidshealth.net

Mental Health America (formerly known as National Mental Health Association)
2000 N. Beauregard Street, 6th Floor
Alexandria, Virginia 22311
Phone: 703-684-7722
Phone: (toll free) 1-800-969-6642
Website: www.nmha.org

Mental Health Matters
P.O. Box 82149
Kenmore, Washington 98028
Phone: 425-402-6934
Website: www.mental-health-matters.com

Mental Health Sanctuary
Website: www.mhsanctuary.com

Mental Health Services Locator
Substance Abuse and Mental Health Services Administration
(SAMHSA)
Website: www.samhsa.gov

Mental Help Net
Website: www.mentalhelp.net
National Alliance on Mental Illness (NAMI)
Colonial Place Three
2107 Wilson Boulevard, Suite 300
Arlington, Virginia 22201
Phone: 703-524-7600
Phone: (toll-free) 1-800-950-6264
Website: www.nami.org

National Association of Anorexia Nervosa and Associated
Disorders (ANAD)
P. O. Box 7
Highland Park, Illinois 60035
Hotline: 847-831-3438
Phone: 847-433-3996
Website: www.anad.org

National Child Abuse Hotline
Phone: (toll-free) 1-800-4-A-CHILD

National Child Advocacy Center (NCAC)
210 Pratt Avenue
Huntsville, Alabama 35801
Phone: 256-533-5437
Website: www.nationalcac.org

National Institute of Mental Health (NIMH)
6001 Executive Boulevard, Room 8184, MSC 9663
Bethesda, Maryland 20892-9663
Phone: (toll-free) 1-866-615-6464
Website: www.nimh.nih.gov

National Teen Dating Abuse Hotline
Phone: (toll-free) 1-866-331-9474
Phone: (toll-free) TTY 1-866-331-8453
Website: www.loveisrespect.org

National Drug Information Treatment and Referral Hotline
Phone: (toll-free) 1-800-662-4357

National Mental Health Consumers' Self-Help Clearing House
1211 Chestnut Street, Suite 1207
Philadelphia, Pennsylvania 19107
Phone: 215-751-1810
Phone: (toll-free) 1-800-553-4539
Website: www.mhselfhelp.org

National Runaway Switchboard
3080 N. Lincoln Avenue
Chicago, Illinois 60657
Phone: 773-880-9860
Phone: (toll-free) 1-800-786-2929
Website: www.1800runaway.org

National Sexual Assault Hotline
Rape, Abuse & Incest National Network
2000 L Street N.W., Suite 406
Washington, D.C. 20036
Phone: 202-544-1034
Phone: (toll-free) 1-800-656-4673 (crisis line)
Website: www.rainn.com

National Suicide Prevention Lifeline
Phone: (toll-free) 1-800-273-8255

National Youth Crisis Hotline
Phone: (toll-free) 1-800-442-4673

Planned Parenthood Federation of America
434 West 33rd Street
New York, NY 10001
Phone: 212-541-7800
Website: www.plannedparenthood.org

Rape, Abuse & Incest National Network (RAINN)
2000 L Street N.W., Suite 406
Washington, DC 20036
Phone: (toll-free) 1-800-656-4673 (crisis line)
Website: www.rainn.org

Substance Abuse and Mental Health Services Administration (SAMHSA)
United States Department of Health and Human Services
Website: http:/www.samhsa.gov

Therapist Locator
Website: www.therapistlocator.net

Treatment Advocacy Center
200 N. Glebe Road, Suite 730
Arlington, Virginia 22203
Phone: 703-294-6001 or 703-294-6002
Website: www.treatmentadvocacycenter.org

WebMD
Website: www.webmd.com

Youth Psych
Website www.youthpsych.com

Comments about The Forgotten Future, are always welcomed and
may be sent to the author
at
P.O. Box 10873
Norfolk, Virginia 23513

Please visit the author's website
at
www.debebel.com

and the author's blog
at
www.forgottenfuture.wordpress.com

www.ingramcontent.com/pod-product-compliance
Lightning Source LLC
Chambersburg PA
CBHW022351280326
41935CB00007B/152